*Fall*osophy

ARDRA SHEPHARD

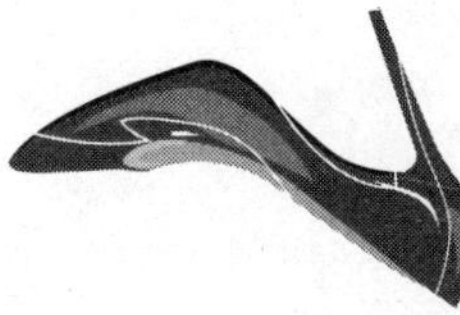

Fall-osophy

My Trip through Life with MS

A MEMOIR

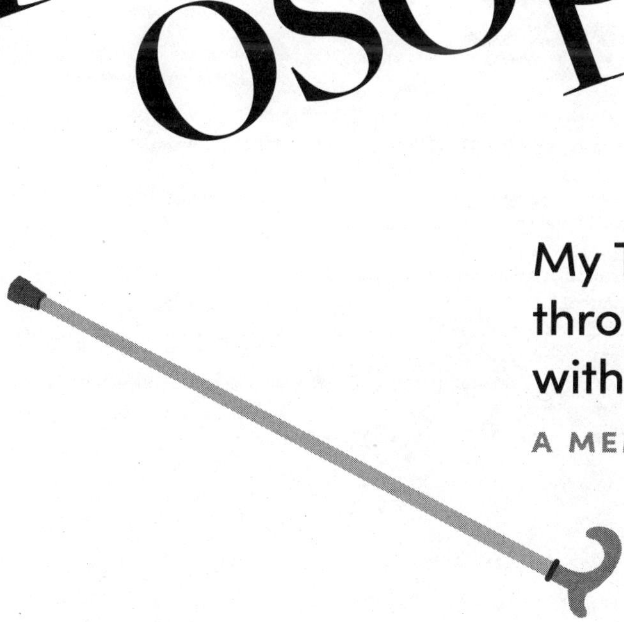

Douglas & McIntyre

1 2 3 4 5 29 28 27 26 25

Douglas and McIntyre (2013) Ltd.
P.O. Box 219, Madeira Park, BC, VON 2HO
www.douglas-mcintyre.com

Edited by Ariel Brewster
Cover artwork by Rachel Joanis
Cover and text design by Naomi MacDougall | DSGN Dept.
Printed and bound in Canada
Printed on 100 percent recycled paper

Canada Council for the Arts | Conseil des Arts du Canada | British Columbia Arts Council | British Columbia
Supported by the Province of British Columbia

Douglas and McIntyre acknowledges the support of the Canada Council for the Arts, the Government of Canada, and the Province of British Columbia through the BC Arts Council.

Library and Archives Canada Cataloguing in Publication

Title: Fallosophy : my trip through life with MS / Ardra Shephard.
Names: Shephard, Ardra, author.
Identifiers: Canadiana (print) 20240504119 | Canadiana (ebook) 20240504127 | ISBN 9781771624305 (softcover) | ISBN 9781771624312 (EPUB)
Subjects: LCSH: Shephard, Ardra. | LCSH: Multiple sclerosis—Patients—Canada—Biography. | LCGFT: Autobiographies.
Classification: LCC RC377 .S54 2025 | DDC 616.8/340092—dc23

For all the Darcys who still believe life is beautiful, and for Kari B., who makes it so.

Contents

For storytelling's sake, some names and identifying details
have been tweaked to protect the innocent and the guilty, and,
most importantly, to protect me (from any awkward phone calls).

1 / Dear Satan

I DON'T EXACTLY BELIEVE in witchcraft, but I'm open to a free consultation. I light more candles than is safe considering the fake cobwebs that overwhelm my already cobwebby apartment. My girlfriends sit in a circle on the living room floor, laughing and chewing on candy necklaces. They're dressed in miniskirts, high heels and heavy makeup, their cowboy hats and cat-ear headbands barely qualifying their skimpy outfits as costumes. It's Halloween and we're about to hit the club where The Bartender works, but first we pre-game over several bottles of red wine, not caring that it's a Tuesday. I dim the lights and join the coven, opening a book of hocus-pocus incantations I picked up I don't even know where.

I look for spells that might fix my life, like *Double, double toil and trouble, release me from the corporate hustle. In the cauldron's bubbling moan, boil and bake my student loan. Fire burn in all its splendour, why am I sleeping with a bartender? Lizard's leg and owlet's wing, somebody clean my apartment.*

It's not our intention to ask the underworld for anything truly evil. We're just looking for a few shortcuts that will make us skinny, improve our credit and give our enemies acne. Unfortunately, the book of spells turns out to be useless. All we can find are some Glinda the Good Witch meditations that promise to release negativity through the power of visualization. I definitely bought it at an Indigo in the suburbs and not on the dark web.

We do a round of shots and make up our own spells. We give up on potions because all I have in my pantry is table salt and a half-eaten box of Froot Loops. Plus, I don't have a cauldron. I don't even have a soup pot. In fact, I have only one pot and it's just big enough to heat up a can of Zoodles. Never mind that it's not even clean right now (I also don't own a dishwasher). I could ask my neighbours if they have any eye of newt, but I wouldn't know where to find a lizard's leg. I'm not sure what an owlet is, but I'm pretty sure it's endangered.

My friends and I may not be competent witches, but intent matters, and our objectives weren't exactly innocent. A few weeks later I will think back to that drunken night and consider that my attempted conversation with the underworld and the shady deals I tried to strike with the Prince of Darkness somehow led to my diagnosis. Random shit doesn't just happen. Bad things happen to bitchy people, and it couldn't just be terrible luck that I'd gotten MS. There had to have been a reason, and for a few years, I will believe the reason is me.

2 / The Before

I SLINK INTO THE OFFICE. Late. I'm in a touched-up version of last night's makeup, so I'm counting on my fresh-from-the-cleaners blazer to make me look pulled together. My left eye hurts in what feels like a hyper-localized, concentrated third-degree hangover. I throw back two Tylenol and take a long sip of the extra-large coffee I've been hiding behind my oversized bag. This isn't the kind of workplace you can saunter into after 9 a.m. flaunting the fact that you made time to stop at Starbucks.

I pass The Bartender—by day he's just another office minion, like me. He carries a leather briefcase, but his soul patch and tight shirts hint at his after-hours gig slinging drinks three nights a week. We nod benign good mornings, like we haven't just seen each other naked.

Approaching my cubicle, I see the phone light up before I hear the quiet trill that is currently my least favourite sound. It's the head micromanager, my boss. He wants to see me in the corporate anteroom. I check my watch: 9:12 a.m. It doesn't matter that I worked until 7 p.m. last night. I'm being summoned to the principal's office. I take one last sip of coffee before I make my way along a cult-y row of cold cubicles and motivational posters encouraging me to "Believe and Succeed."

My security pass doesn't give me access to the executive wing and I have to be buzzed in like a nobody. There aren't any posters here; it's all original art, exotic fish and textured upholstery. The lobby houses two parrots—the bougie, talking kind. The anteroom smells like synthetic vanilla and feels like a more expensive version of the "good" living room your grandmother never uses.

I steel myself for another lecture about how my workday starts at 8:55. But Big Boss greets me with a warm smile instead. The company would like to offer me a promotion. The dot-com boom is driving growth and they need someone who speaks French to *blah blah blah*. The details don't matter. I'm getting a bonus and a raise. I'm even getting an award for the work I've been doing. For some reason, Colin Powell will be at the ceremony, and I can tell by the way Big Boss says "Colin Powell" that I should be impressed, or at least know who the hell Colin Powell is. (*Does he work here?*) I can bring two guests, which will obviously be my parents. Unless there's an open bar, there's no way my friends would sit through speeches just to watch me get a prize I don't deserve for doing my non-sports-related job in suburban Southern Ontario.

I'm not remotely qualified to work in finance. It's not imposter syndrome. I am an imposter. I live in my overdraft and still use my fingers for basic math. I don't have a business degree. I haven't even finished my arts degree. This gig was only ever supposed to be a placeholder. An income until my real life starts. I don't want a future in this fluorescent-lit corporate purgatory, though it does feel good to be recognized? I try to hide my surprise but Big Boss clocks it. He tells me I'm smart and that management sees my potential. He calls me a "real up-and-comer." He puts his hand on my shoulder and tells me in a don't-fuck-it-up tone of voice that from now on my day starts at 8 a.m.

On my way back to my cubicle, I stop at my best friend Tracy's desk to see if she can give me a handful of Advil. The Tylenol hasn't kicked in, my eye is throbbing and I figure I must have more of an ibuprofen hangover than an acetaminophen one. While she searches her purse, I spill the news that five minutes earlier I'd promised to keep confidential. She's less impressed than I thought she'd be. "Don't get attached to the money. It's a trap that will keep you from getting out of here. Let's hit the mall after work and set that pay bump on fire."

I do want out of this confining cubicle and out of this boring town. The worst possible future for me is an ordinary one. The idea of a minivan, a picket fence and buying groceries from Costco to feed my two and a half kids gives me hives. I want to see the world, to live in cosmopolitan cities surrounded by creative people and original thinkers. I'm determined to live a life of excitement, of purpose, of dreams.

More specifically, I want to be the next Maria Callas (minus a smooth-talking Onassis, of course). When I'm forced to work late, I sing scales in the bathroom. I can't afford to go back to school to study opera properly. I don't have enough disposable income to blow on private lessons with a top singing teacher either, but that is exactly what I do. Every Saturday

I write a probably bad cheque for seventy-five dollars and make my way from Hamilton to north of Toronto. It takes me two and a half hours on a bus, a train, a subway and another bus to get to my teacher's studio. I get a hot dog from the street vendor between the GO station and the subway, because I am not an adult. I spend rent money on private acting lessons from a sketchy out-of-work actor and grocery money on headshots (and let's face it, vodka shots), but none of it is enough. Nobody becomes an opera singer in Hamilton; I don't care how many Italians live here.

I have a dream, but I don't have a plan. I'm twenty-three; I still have time to make mistakes and figure my shit out. At least, I think I do.

WEEKS LATER, MY EYE has not stopped hurting and I'm forced to admit it's not a hangover. Maybe I got something stuck in there? Can migraines live in your eye? It's okay if I look straight ahead, but if I move my eye even slightly, it feels like I'm being stabbed. This is especially problematic because rolling my eyes is an essential communication skill that I'm unwilling to abandon.

I'd convinced myself that whatever's going on with my eye would eventually go away on its own, but on the day of the award ceremony, where I am to be celebrated by God and Colin Powell himself, it's not just pain—my eye now feels like it's coated in Vaseline. I rub away the blurriness, but I can hardly see. I curse myself for not having replaced my mascara since the 1990s, but for some reason, even my cursing doesn't sound right. I curse again, louder, and realize my hearing is muffled in my right ear. *What the fuck.* This is incredibly inconvenient. Obviously I don't have a migraine. It must be a sinus infection or the flu, and I don't have time for the fucking flu. I'm getting an award and I have yet to google Colin Powell.

I walk from my Westdale apartment to the emergency room at Hamilton's McMaster hospital (Mac), resigned to the fact that I'm going to have to hang around for hours just to get some antibiotics. Smart phones have yet to be invented and texting is still in its infancy; it's like banging out Morse code on my flip phone. Not worth it. There's nothing but old issues of *Canadian Living* and *Chatelaine* to peruse with my "good" eye, and the anxiety of possibly missing the award ceremony, to keep me occupied.

My blood is collected, I have a CT scan and I indignantly pee in a cup, as if something in my urine could possibly have anything in common with vision loss. It all feels like overkill. I'm passed around between nurses and technicians for hours until I finally meet with the doctor, like he's the Wizard of Oz. He turns out to be a gentle and sympathetic older man who tells me all these tests are to rule out the bad stuff. I take him at his word. I have no reason not to. Later, I will remember his kindness. I will realize he knew.

Finally, I'm released and told to come back the next day to see a neurologist. I'm more annoyed than alarmed—I don't want to spend another day in a waiting room, but I don't have time to protest. I don't even have time for makeup and a wardrobe change. The Bartender collects me and we arrive at the award ceremony just as it's starting. It's November 27, 2000, and the US presidential election is being contested. Colin Powell opens with a joke about not knowing if he will be the next secretary of state or not *(oh, he's a politician)* before launching into his speech about children and education or something else inspiring. Meanwhile, I have roughly fourteen hours of my own precious ignorance left.

MY MOM INSISTS on coming to my appointment with the neurologist. I didn't ask her to be here, but I guess she wants to hang out. When the nurse calls my name, I leave my mom in the waiting room, because I have no idea that my life is about to implode.

I'm asked about symptoms I've never had. I'm forced to pee in a cup, again. I'm subjected to increasingly bizarre tests, including a "touch my finger, touch your nose, close your eyes and turn yourself around" hokey-pokey that makes me wonder if I'm being punked. When the doctor opens a safety pin and drags the sharp end across the bottom of my bare foot, I start to think med school must not be as hard as I've been led to believe.

When the exam is over, the lights don't dim, music doesn't start to play. Nobody takes my hand or says, "I think you'd better sit down." Granted, I am already sitting, but there is no warning about the bomb that's about to be dropped. I'm completely unprepared when the doctor unceremoniously declares, "You have optic neuritis and there's a 50 percent chance you have multiple sclerosis. MS."

My stomach turns itself inside out and my heartbeat relocates to my face. I have no idea what optic neuritis is, and, in fact, refer to it as optic neurosis the first fifty times I say it. As for MS, I know only it's bad—catastrophic, despite the doctor's confoundingly neutral tone. I find no comfort in the fifty-fifty odds Dr. Poker Face has given me. I skip right past denial and start to cry so hard I can't catch my breath. The doctor leaves without closing the door behind him. My meltdown isn't private, but I am alone.

Eventually a nurse sticks her head in and asks if I want her to get my mom, as if this isn't obvious. When my mom arrives, she has not been briefed. I am angry that I have to deliver the news to her myself—I'm the one who has to tell my mother her daughter might have MS.

Norma takes the news more calmly than I do. She typically has a "what do they know?" and "who do they think they are?" kind of attitude to most authorities, and immediately latches on to the 50 percent possibility that it is not, in fact, MS. It's a very on-brand response for a woman whose guiding principles include a combination of optimism and wilful ignorance of unpleasant information. I'm not convinced or soothed. I'm not prone to assuming the worst, but I can't get past the sickening feeling that this is real, that this is happening.

While we wait for the results of an MRI, it's a surreal seven weeks of knowing that MS is a threat but not a guarantee. People tell me they're praying for me, as if there's still time to change what has already been set in motion. My family expresses relief that a diagnosis won't ruin Christmas. A friend insists that pretty people don't get MS. Big Boss assures me I can't possibly have MS because the Good Lord wouldn't let something like this happen to someone like me. I am inundated with the conviction of those around me that MS simply isn't an option.

By the time my follow-up appointment comes around, I've developed numbness in my toes and on parts of my face. I've been losing my balance and I can't seem to walk in a straight line. I've spent enough time on the internet that I don't need test results to know that I for sure have MS. When Dr. Poker Face shows me the six white spots on my MRI that confirm the diagnosis, I crack a joke. On some level, I already have a sense that one of the burdens of being sick forever is to let others know I'm okay.

3 / Welcome to Brain Damage

IT'S A GREY, COLOURLESS DAY when my mom and I leave the hospital. The weather matches my mood and I feel grateful the universe didn't ruin sunny days for me—January 11 was always going to be a day you didn't mind wrecking.

My dad picks us up in his minivan and my mom insists I take the front seat. My new sick-person status has already changed the dynamic of how I am to be treated. I'm delicate now.

"Well, it's MS," I tell my dad in the chillest, I've-got-this tone of voice available to me. He breathes a sigh of relief, like this is good news. It's not a brain tumour. I'm annoyed. I'm being brave here. It's not a brain tumour but it's certainly not nothing! Brain tumour was never a contender for What's Wrong with Ardra anyway, and even if it had been, MS hardly feels like a consolation prize. I've already decided I don't want to be pitied, but it would be nice to pour one out for the old me before people who are *not* me start looking for silver linings.

I start leafing through the glossy pamphlets I was given by the MS clinic. The brochures feature impossibly happy people and phrases like "MS Lives Here" that belie the information they're trying to communicate—that MS attacks the brain and spinal cord, that it can be severely disabling, that it's a condition without a cure. And, fair enough, "Welcome to Brain Damage" wouldn't look good on a pamphlet, but these stupid smiling people don't seem to appreciate how bad their disease is. I read out loud from a list of possible symptoms printed in cheerful fonts about what my not-a-brain-tumour disease might gift me. Bladder incontinence. Bowel incontinence. What the hell is sexual dysfunction?

My dad drives on in silence.

I've been diagnosed with relapsing remitting multiple sclerosis, or RRMS. A chronic progressive disease intent on destroying my central nervous system, or CNS. *Chronic* means "forever" and *progressive* means "it gets worse." CNS means the thing that basically runs the show. The good news is, I'm not always going to feel as weak and as blind as I do right now. The first *R* of RRMS means that my current symptoms are being caused by a relapse, also known as an attack. My cannibal body's immune system is chewing on my myelin sheath—the protective coating of my nerves—and leaving me with something like a frayed electrical cord that keeps my nerves from transmitting clear signals. The second *R* of this fucked-up alphabet soup means that over the next couple of months this attack should resolve. But *remission* is kind of a bullshit term, because every attack can leave a bit of damage. Eventually my ability to recover from these assaults will start to wane. *FML* means "fuck my life."

My dad drops my mom and me off at my second-storey one-bedroom Westdale walk-up. It's the first place I've ever lived that was all my own. It's messy and lacks closet space. A rotating pile of designer clothes I can't afford takes up half the real estate on my queen-sized bed. I never cook, but the kitchen smells vaguely like garlic. I didn't paint when I moved in. The bedroom is a deep pumpkin and the living room is forest green. High-drama colours appeal to me, but I wouldn't have chosen these shades myself. The living room still has the battered cat-scratched leather sofa and loveseat I paid fifty bucks for when the previous tenant didn't want to move them. I'm too busy and too broke to spend money fixing things that are good enough. I haven't made this apartment my own because I didn't think I was supposed to be here long-term. Nothing about my squatter life is supposed to be permanent. Except now, MS. MS officially belongs to me, even if it feels like the opposite is true. MS is the first immutable thing I get to know about my grown-up life.

The group text hasn't been invented yet—in 2001 we still talk on the phone. I set my mom up with a list of people who are waiting for an update and the land line in my bedroom while I hide in the next room trying to talk myself out of eavesdropping as she tells my friends, one by one, that I have MS. I know I'm being dramatic. My MS might be official now but the diagnosis itself is only a shock to the holdouts who refused to believe it could happen.

It's not that I can't bear to say the words "I have MS," it's that I don't have the energy to respond to any *rah, rah, you got this* cheerleading bullshit. *If anyone can handle MS, it's you!* As if MS is some kind of reward for being strong. And why does everyone think I'm strong anyway? I'm mouthy and extroverted and opinionated. Being bossy and a little entitled hasn't exactly prepared me to take on paralysis.

I need my friends to say: "This sucks. How is it that you're even prettier when you're crying? Let's get fucked up when you're ready." But I can't risk it. I have a sense that every detail of this day is being seared into my long-term memory, and I've already heard enough things I'll never un-hear for one day.

The Bartender is the only person I actually want to see. When he shows up, I describe my day in gossipy detail, trying to keep things light. I roll my eyes (fucking ouch) when I tell him how someone from St. Luke's, a local church where I am sometimes hired to sing, told my mom they're taking me off the prayer list now that I've been diagnosed. I tell him that Dr. Poker Face's office is painted My Little Pony pink. I tell him I had an avocado sandwich for lunch—that it was just okay, that it would have been better if they'd left it in the panini press for thirty seconds longer. I laugh when I tell him about the nurse I've already decided to hate. She has an attitude of resignation and dresses like a kindergarten teacher. In her ankle-skimming knock-off Laura Ashley frock, even her wardrobe is patronizing. When The Bartender suggests I might be experiencing a shoot-the-messenger mentality, I don't disagree, but I do double down. Maybe it's not Maryanna's fault I have MS, but *something* is her fault and I'm gonna be low-key hostile to her until I figure it out. I laugh again when I tell him my eighteen-year-old brother James worried I was contagious, as if any of this is funny. I recap my day like it was a normal, if somewhat quirky Thursday.

I don't tell him about the pamphlets.

I barely notice that The Bartender doesn't have much to say. It's not unusual for me to do 70 percent of the talking. Eighty if I've got news and the headlines are all mine today. What I don't say is that I've decided I'm not going to let my diagnosis change the dynamics of our relationship. Of any of my relationships. I've resolved to face this disease, stand up to it, not let it stop me. It's my first official day with MS and I'm determined to live my life the same way I always thought I would, without concessions. I don't want to be disabled. So I decide I won't be. As if it's up to me.

The Bartender kisses me good night and I end his hug early. I haven't cried all day, but I know that if I let myself sink into him, I will break. He leaves in an unprecedented *I'm-not-even-gonna-try-to-have-sex-with-you* kind of way. I pretend not to notice, but it's unnerving.

4 / Drop and Flop

I DON'T KNOW WHAT to expect from my MS, but it seems like there should be an urgent list of disease stuff to do now that it's official. When I ask Dr. Poker Face if there are any medications I should be on, he says, "Are you rich?" Uhm, no? He tells me that the meds that treat MS start at forty thousand. A year. And if I have a job with benefits, I'd better not quit. Ever. This is an objectively horrifying development, but I can only process one calamity at a time.

Dr. Poker Face hands me four pamphlets and tells me to read them over and let him know which medication I would prefer, like I'm the one who went to med school. He tells me that "early intervention" is key, so I expect to leave with a prescription, but "early intervention" belongs solidly between those sarcastic quotation marks. MS treatment lives in its own time zone. Eastern Chronic Whenever the Fuck We Feel Like It Time is dictated by an under-resourced health-care system that can be slow to diagnose MS and insurance companies that seem pretty chill about getting to you when they get to you. Try not to worry about your untreated brain damage in the meantime.

The upside to all this medical inefficiency is that I'm free to go on the non-refundable beach vacay I booked with The Bartender back when I believed only suckers paid for cancellation insurance. I was younger and stupider back in mid-November, before my sophisticated new vocabulary included words like *myelin sheath*, *interferon* and *oligoclonal bands*. Two months ago I would have assumed *Lhermitte's* was a high-end department store. *Spinal tap* was just a stupid stoner movie. I'm still not sure what *evoked potentials* are, but I'm pretty sure I'm wasting them.

So, yeah. I could use a vacation.

It's the first time either The Bartender or I have been to an all-inclusive resort and I discover that it's possible to be happy, or at least happy-adjacent, even when my world is in turmoil. After an unremarkable flight, a coach bus delivers us from the airport to a massive open-air marble lobby where we are greeted with watered-down cocktails and cool face cloths. It feels classy the way small courtesies do when you're twenty-three and someone calls your boyfriend "sir." We spend seven days pointing, slack-jawed, at the free-range flamingos wandering the property. We take pictures with disposable cameras of the ice-sculptured fish on the buffet table and the towel swans on our beds as if Instagram had already been invented. The Bartender buys me a bracelet that we are assured is of the finest quality silver and topaz. We sample rum and purchase as much as we are legally permitted to bring back to Canada, because we're convinced we've never had better than Brugal. Considering our palates were weaned on Malibu and whatever rum they put in rum and coke when you order one at the club, our assessment is probably accurate.

We take full advantage of "all-inclusive." We're not keen on getting up early, but we don't want to miss out on all-you-can-eat bacon either. Determined to sample as many of the blended drinks as possible, we consult the sticky laminated menu multiple times a day to gauge our progress. We are in rapture of the nightly live shows. We can't believe the quality of the knock-off Cirque du Soleil performers and the Michael Jackson impersonator. We are impressed by everything.

My eyesight is still wonky, so The Bartender walks with me and patiently explains every item at the buffet in excruciating detail. I can't complain, because he is being thoughtful, but the process is tedious and tiring and I don't really care if I have pink watermelon or yellow. In general, The Bartender and I do not have the same decision-making style. I am quick and decisive, sometimes impulsive. I trust my gut and will happily roll the dice and pick a book or a movie by its cover. Renting a movie with The Bartender means I need to clear my schedule. This dude needs to read the back of every box and consider all his options. He narrows shit down and asks the staff for recommendations that he will then ignore. A trip to the video store with The Bartender means contemplating every title from action to indie until your clothes start to smell like free popcorn and imitation butter. The way you do anything is the way you do everything and The Bartender brings his Blockbuster Video MO to the buffet table.

We hold up the line a handful of times before The Bartender starts to notice that it's actually pretty exhausting for me to spend so much time on my feet. I'm relieved when he offers to make me a plate. The Bartender has dedicated himself to making sure I'm comfortable and have everything I need. I reluctantly accept this level of attention. This trip is my chance to prove I'm still me. Still fun and cool, not high maintenance, and I'm already concerned that I'm failing.

When I need a break from worrying about what will happen to my body, I switch gears to worry about who will love me now. After my diagnosis, a friend thought they were saying something helpful and told me that it's a good thing I'm single because whoever I marry will "know what they're getting into." Like I'm damaged goods. I can't help but wonder if I will have to settle for some second-tier mouth breather or if I will be forced to reassess how I feel about cats. I'm not sure what my situationship with a twenty-eight-year-old club kid who hasn't left the nest is exactly, but now is not the time to figure it out. We're not here to figure anything out, at least not together. We don't talk about our relationship. We never have. So we don't talk about MS either.

I'm lying by the pool giving myself random vision tests, closing one eye and seeing if I can still make out the same blurry objects I could yesterday. I want to read but I'm struggling to get through the only book I brought with me, a large-print edition of a memoir by a woman with MS. The author makes it sound like MS is no big deal and it all feels kind of phony. The book is heavy on being inspiring (barf) and heavy in general. Why are large-print books all hardcover? I'm sweaty and it's making the book jacket slide against my bare leg. I've been baking in the heat for a couple of hours and I need to pee.

I scan the area around the pool for a blurry outline of someone tall and thin. The Bartender left to get pina coladas a while ago, and he should be back by now. I need him to help direct me to the outdoor bathroom. I can probably figure it out, but I have to get really close to the sign to tell if I'm going into the room for *hombres* or *mujeres*. Plus, it helps to have his arm to steady me. I'm a bit more off-balance the last couple of days. My 11 a.m. gait looks as drunk as the gait of the actual day drinkers, the hardcore crew with the leathery backs who sit at the swim-up bar all day and don't bother to get out of the pool to pee.

The Bartender is still MIA when suddenly my need to pee has escalated from a nice-to-have into something that's happening whether I want it to or not. I'm going to have to wing it and walk to the bathroom on my own. If I end up in the wrong *baño*, so be it.

I reach for my flip-flops but my torso doesn't follow. That's weird. I try to sit up again and I can't. What the actual fuck. I use my arms to shimmy myself up from my lounger into a sitting position. My inner panic button is unsure whether to be more freaked out about sudden paralysis or my desperate need to pee.

"What's wrong?" The Bartender is back. Finally. The look on my face is clearly communicating agitation.

"Uhm, no biggie, I just have to pee. Also, it's kind of hard to get up?" He bends down and helps me stand. I need a lot of support as we do a slow walk to the bathroom. Nobody thought to warn me that heat can exacerbate MS symptoms, that even a half-degree increase in body temperature can slow down nerve conduction and make you feel like you're having an attack. Heat can fuck up MS so badly that before we had sophisticated magnets to take a peek inside the skull, MS was diagnosed with a "hot bath" test. Which is exactly what it sounds like, except so antiquated I can't help but wonder if they offered the exam as part of a "find out if she's a witch" package deal.

By the time we make it to the bathroom, I am grateful to be wearing a bikini bottom, and "make it" is a generous assessment of events. I've leaked a bit, but I don't think it's noticeable. It's not even enough to bring some relief; I still have to pee like I've never had to pee before. Still, the leak is shocking. I can Kegel like an Olympian and this came out of nowhere. When I finally collapse on the public toilet, I don't even care that the seat is wet with pool water. I am so relieved to be sitting and to have narrowly escaped humiliation. I look forward to the satisfied feeling of an empty bladder. We made it. Mostly. Close enough. *We're safe now*, I tell my bladder. *Time to let go*.

But nothing happens. My bladder confoundingly refuses to empty.

SIX DAYS IN, neither one of us knows what to do about my sudden decline. We make an appointment with our designated travel rep, a perky expat living the dream selling day trips to tourists and hooking up with locals while she dodges her student loans and heals from her divorce. (I assume.) We need someone in authority to tell us what to do, and Starla is the closest option to someone in charge in a country that suddenly feels very foreign.

Starla confirms that there's a resort doctor on call, but that he mostly treats minor cuts and UTIs. She's pretty sure active brain damage is beyond his purview. After seeing me walk, Starla tells me she will arrange for a wheelchair to meet me at the airport. We're going home tomorrow. I feel relief and horror. It wouldn't have occurred to me that airport wheelchair service even exists, let alone that it would be available to someone like me. This isn't my world. Except it is.

For the rest of the trip, The Bartender never takes his eyes off of me. He seems to know when I want to move and is ready with an arm to steady me. I'm not completely incapacitated. We still lounge by the pool, play cards and go to the shows. We're still having sex. But it's not the same. My whole body feels foreign to me. Like I've been Freaky Friday'd and I'm existing in someone else's skin, waiting for lightning to strike and put me back in my own anatomy.

The Bartender has taken good care of me, but back in Canada, he drops me off at my parents' place looking visibly relieved. My mom invites him to come in and have a drink, but he declines. Like an under-qualified babysitter handing back a kid they had no idea was an uncontrolled pyromaniac, he can't get away fast enough. I can't blame him. He signed up for a sexy beach vacay, not an unpaid internship as a personal care worker. I didn't exactly nail fun, cool and low maintenance, but I have bigger things to worry about.

5 / There's No Place Like Home

THE NEXT MORNING, I'm back at Mac before I've even had a chance to unpack. I hand a nurse my urine sample and she explains that bladder infections can jack up MS symptoms. It seems sketchy: like, how does a UTI make you fall down? But just like the sun can elevate body temperature and fuck up nerve conduction, a fever or an infection can exacerbate MS symptoms. The result is what's known as a pseudo relapse. A temporary MS fake-out.

Once a UTI is ruled out, I can be treated for what this actually is: a full-blown real-ass relapse. I'm hooked up to an IV and given a dose of steroids so high it comes with a warning: I will not be myself. My first experience with Solu-Medrol isn't addictive in the medical sense but it is intoxicating. By the end of the day, my walking and vision are dramatically better. The high I get from how much easier it suddenly is to walk and see is a dragon I will chase for the next twenty years.

Meanwhile, I finally feel like someone is doing something about my out-of-control disease and I ask why the eff I wasn't given this magic potion three months ago when I first showed up half-blind. I'm told that steroids can improve symptoms temporarily, but they don't influence long-term outcomes—once an MS attack runs its course, the amount of damage it leaves behind is the same as it would have been with or without steroids.

I have a hard time accepting that a drug that has had such a profound and immediate impact on my relapse could have any downside. Of course, I will soon learn that if something seems too good to be true, it's probably gonna give you acne. It's definitely going to give you pie-face, next-level hiccups and insomnia. I'm too scared to google "buffalo hump" and nobody tells me that by the time I'm forty I'll have full-fledged osteo-fucking-porosis. Still, steroids seem worth it. There's no high like the high of being able to walk after a period of paralysis. I assume. I mean, I haven't actually tried heroin.

Dr. Poker Face tells me to take some time off. No working for two or three months, no singing lessons. My job is to rest. It's a shocking amount of time, but I'm grateful for the directive. I don't know what I'm doing or how I'm supposed to feel. I don't know how much I'm supposed to power through. Nothing makes sense.

I'm not even going back to my apartment just yet. Nobody thinks I should be alone anyway. I could pull myself up the stairs to the second floor, but there are three floating steps in front of my building that have no railing, and without a railing I might as well be trying to scale Everest without a Sherpa or do math without a calculator. (Later, I will ask my Westdale slumlord not for a railing—I wouldn't want to put anyone out—but for some kind of stake in the ground next to the steps, just so I could have something to grab on to. She will say no and I will have to move.)

The drive from Mac to my parents' house in neighbouring Burlington seems long, like I'm driving away from my old life, my former self. Burlington, which is right next door to Hamilton but far enough from Toronto to lack meaningful diversity or pizza that's not from a chain, still considers itself a city. But Burlington is not a *city*-city. There's no orchestra, no interesting architecture. It's the kind of place where Swiss Chalet makes the Top Ten Restaurants on Tripadvisor. Sure, there are trees, baseball diamonds, a lake. You can feed baby ducks in the spring. You're probably not going to get murdered. You decide if a craft store the size of a school gymnasium is a good or a bad thing. Burlington is home to Canada's largest Ribfest, when every August a four-day cloud of smoke hovers over the entire city (again, your call on whether this is a pro or a con). Burlington is the burbs. "The 905." And I am allergic to the burbs.

My parents' house, though, isn't even in the burbs—my mom and dad live in the country. Where horror movies are set. There are no neighbours, no corner store, no corners. Right on the edge of town, their street doesn't even have a name—it's just a numbered side road, a placeholder, until the municipality decides No. 2 is worth baptizing.

I don't complain (I do). My life is on hold while I spend the next three months with my parents, fighting cabin fever, trying not to regress to my teenage self, recovering from this attack. It's a relief not to have to think about anything. I don't have to make the bed, or dinner, or even the smallest decisions. There's only one TV and it will not occur to my dad to ask me what I want to watch.

My mom is ready to mother me, even if she's in active denial. She's convinced that her beloved chiropractor and the baby Jesus can fix whatever I've got going on. In the meantime, she's eager to indulge me. Do I want her heirloom jewellery? A homemade pie? If she could shop or bake or gift her way to curing me, she would.

When we arrive, there's a delivery of medical supplies waiting at the door of my parents' house. It's all the gear the nurse who's coming for the next four days will need to administer the rest of my steroids. Nothing says "haunted house" quite like an IV pole on the front porch. I feel like I'm in a movie.

It's hard to believe I was in the Dominican Republic just yesterday. After an epically long day at the hospital, I'm ready for the longest sleep of my life. Unfortunately, there's a heparin lock in my arm to keep my vein open for the duration of my infusions and I worry about how I'll manage to sleep without dislodging the tube and bleeding out in the night. I build a pillow fort around my arm and tell my subconscious we're sleeping on our back this week, no turning. I spend the next few days skipping showers for fear of bloodstream infection.

When the nurse runs the IV drip too quickly, my arm starts to throb. The steroids enter my body through my bloodstream but they fill my mouth with the taste of metal. I try to chase it away with ginger ale and hard candies, but it's no use. The poison is coming from inside the house.

When my five-day treatment is over, The Bartender takes me to the movies—my first time leaving my parents' house since the hospital, my first time seeing anyone other than Jim and Norma, my brother James and the nurse. When we get to the multiplex, I practically float up the dozen or so stairs outside the building. Showing off, I exclaim, "Did you see that?" I walk back down the stairs and then up again. "No hands! No railing!" The Bartender acts impressed but not blown away. Almost as if he's humouring me, like I'm a six-year-old doing a poorly executed cartwheel. The Bartender isn't prone to big emotions, but I feel like he should be more pumped about my Lazarus-level recovery. Maybe it's just the under-reaction of someone who has never had their ability to walk threatened. Which would be better than what I fear: that he can't erase the version of me he saw on our beach vacation.

IT'S TIME TO start a disease-modifying therapy, or a DMT—a drug. And it's a whole thing. I never want to hear Maryanna's annoying singsong voice again, but I can't dodge the MS clinic any longer. In 2001, DMTs are relatively new in the world of MS care, and I can tell I'm supposed to feel lucky to have access to a drug that might reduce my attacks by one-third—33 percent. Worse still is that the drug I'm prescribed has to be given by needle, three times a week. Hell to the fuck no. Except I can't say no, because even as I learn to expect bruising, welts and flu-like side effects, I know that all of this unpleasantness is still better than what unchecked MS might do.

A new nurse comes to the house to teach me how to shoot up, and yes, I've decided to refer to this process as shooting up. She arrives with an overwhelming amount of drug paraphernalia. I wonder where I'm supposed to store the bulky bright red and yellow sharps container in my little apartment. I don't want to see it. I don't want to be reminded of how fucked all of this is every time I reach under the sink for my hair dryer.

The nurse explains everything in tedious detail. It's a lot to absorb and my attitude about all of it is negative. My mom is a former nurse herself, and she and I already agreed that she will give me my shots until I can summon the courage to take this on myself. But the judgy nurse is unimpressed and refuses to leave until I show her I know how to prep the site, load the auto-injector and fire a test run into my thigh. The auto-injector is supposed to make the process less scary. I press the button and I know it doesn't sound like a *literal* gunshot, but it's a disturbingly loud bang. It still feels scary.

AS MY STRENGTH improves, so does my restlessness. It's hard to go from having every minute accounted for to being accountable to no one. Barbara Walters and Joy Behar don't give a fuck whether or not I show up at eleven for Hot Topics. MS doesn't feel like an emergency anymore and I'm ready to think about cautiously re-entering the land of the living.

My dad drives me to work a handful of times so that I can show my face while I'm recovering and everyone can look at me sideways and with a degree of pity. *That's the girl with MS. The one we made the donation for.* The CEO has a soft spot for me. Not because I'm good at my job, but because I founded and conduct the corporate choir. I even talked him into buying us a piano. He let me pick one out and I chose a seven-foot 1920s Steinway. He sets up a meeting with one of the firm's portfolio managers. Apparently we're heavily invested in a pharmaceutical company with a flagship MS drug. I spend ninety minutes of a big shot's time getting the health-care version of insider trading.

When I meet with HR about what a return to work might look like, the response is a bit cooler. Dana casually tells me that everyone's insurance premiums are going up because of me. I feel like she expects me to say thank you. We make a plan to ease me back into corporate life with reduced hours and yet-to-be-determined modifications to accommodate the inconvenience of my low vision. My job is safe and I feel grateful and lucky, without considering my employer's benevolence-to-legal-obligation ratio.

My parents sit me down. "We would like you to think about moving here," my dad says with a straight face. "Permanently."

"The front living room could be just for you and your guests—private," my mom continues. My eyes are wide. The suggestion is ludicrous. I already know I can't live in this haunted house in the middle of nowhere, but I don't want to seem ungrateful, so I temper my revulsion with reason. I don't have a car. I only recently learned to drive, and I want my five hundred bucks back from Young Drivers because now, thanks to optic neuritis, I may never get my licence.

"I would take you to work," my dad adds. They've got it all worked out. Uber doesn't exist yet. I can't be dependent on my dad to leave what is suddenly starting to feel like a light *Misery* situation.

"You can have gentlemen callers. It's none of our business," Norma says as I swallow my own vomit. Why are they so worried about me? I'm getting better! Why do they think I won't be able to look after myself? (To be fair, my mom's still doing my injections. Not to mention my laundry.)

"Think about it," my dad continues. "You don't have to answer now."

Ribfest and gentlemen callers. This cannot be my future. My parents can't fix this for me, but they can definitely make it worse. My dad is right: It's time to think about what my future with this disease looks like. It's time to figure out a new normal. It's time for me to do my own needles. It's time for me to go home.

6 / Whine Club

I NEED A FRIEND. I'm not looking to replace my existing friends, the ones who've helped me navigate breakups and bullshit work dynamics, who've nursed me through hangovers and talked me out of cutting my own bangs. Tracy can be counted on to hate the same people I hate and when she figured out she hated her boyfriend, she let me practise driving stick on his eighty-thousand-dollar Escalade (hi, John!). My cousin Laura has been looking out for me since high school, when she introduced me to the Smiths and showed me how to roll my Catholic school kilt. She's too principled to help me hide a body, but she's a lawyer now—she knows how to keep a secret.

My friends are here for my MS, but they can't relate to injection site reactions and intermittent paralysis. My friends can cheerlead and champion and tell me "you've got this," but how could they possibly know? I need a friend who understands how to handle this disease or who can at least say, "oh my god, me too." I'm desperate for hard proof that at least one other real-life twenty-something woman is handling MS so that I can believe I can handle it too. I need an MS friend.

I don't yet know it, but MS is so pervasive that it will take only a few years for my world to include colleagues, acquaintances, friends and even family members with MS. It will feel almost impossible to imagine there was ever a time when I felt like I was the only one. Even if I somehow know that a posse of people with MS is in my future, I can't wait for them to trickle into my life. I'm desperate to connect with someone who gets it now.

I've been resisting the MS Society as a resource because MS isn't a club I want to be in and the idea of attending a support group is extremely unappealing. I need an MS friend, but I'm not interested in being part of any recovery-style, group-therapy circle of confession and vulnerability. I'm at least a decade away from even considering there are things I cannot change, let alone accepting them. I'm not looking for serenity. Serenity is for quitters.

Unfortunately, I know that I'm not going to find an MS friend organically—there's no social media in 2001, and a support group feels like my only option. Tracy agrees to come with me—in fact, the support group was her idea.

When we arrive, we are not welcomed so much as scolded.

"No students!" proclaims a woman with a clipboard sitting behind a rickety wooden table, the kind you find in church basements. My back is already up. I'm anxious about being here and I don't have the energy to convince anyone that I have the sick-person secret password. I'm ready to bail, but Tracy pipes up, "We're not students. She has MS."

"Oh, sorry! We get lots of students this time of year. Are you here for the support group, then?" Obviously, but the woman sounds genuinely confused. As we enter the room, I start to understand why.

The Hamilton MS Society chapter is located in a dreary building in the rough part of town. Once inside, I have to remind myself that we're not actually in a basement. The windows are covered with blackout curtains and a layer of dust that suggests the drapes have never been opened. If they're trying to project a "nothing to steal here" atmosphere, it's working, but there's literally nothing to steal, unless you need a commercial-grade coffee urn, or expired Voortman wafers. Even the fake plant looks dead. It's the kind of space that feels designed to encourage resignation. I get it: we can't have these meetings at the Four Seasons (but why?). Surely we can do better than this.

Half a dozen people sit in a wide circle under the hum of the one fluorescent light that's working. Everyone is at least twenty years older and a hundred years sicker than I am. There are wheelchairs, powerchairs—one guy is totally blind. It feels like a horror movie whose working title is *Welcome to Your Bleak Fucking Future.*

"Keep an open mind," Tracy whispers under her breath. "It's just an hour, then we'll go get drunk somewhere."

The group all seems to know each other and nobody pays attention to me or Tracy, until the facilitator who initially tried to turn us away introduces me.

"This is Andra and she was recently diagnosed," she says in a pleading tone, as if she's trying to coax the group to be nice, or to at least humour me.

"Actually, it's Ardra," I correct her.

"Oh, sorry! Ar-Ardra? Am I saying that right?"

"Doesn't matter," says one of the group members. "The young ones never come back."

Rude, but I already know he's right. Nonetheless, I'm here, so I ask my questions.

"So, what drugs are you guys on?" *Nice opener*, I think to myself. I'm definitely not doing anything to diminish any AA energy, but I genuinely want to hear how others are handling side effects. Better still if someone can tell me that the drugs they're on are working to control their MS. My question is popular and the group is suddenly animated, talking about painkillers, antidepressants, sleeping pills, anxiety meds and the occasional upper. There are heavy endorsements of marijuana, which is not yet close to being legal. It's an overwhelming list of pharmaceuticals, and now I feel like we're all to blame for the substance-abuse vibe, but nobody mentions the kinds of drugs I'm interested in.

"Oh, I meant what *disease-modifying drugs* are you on. DMDs?" Crickets. Not one person is on a disease-modifying therapy. Most have never even heard of DMT or DMDs. I am appalled without appreciating how new this class of MS drug therapy is. I don't yet understand that the treatments that are available to people like me, with relapsing MS, are not and have never been available to the people in the room, who almost certainly all have some form of progressive MS. I don't feel particularly lucky, so I don't understand that these people were not as lucky as I am to have been diagnosed at a time when any MS therapies were available at all. Instead, I'm full of judgment as I wonder silently how these people could just sit back and let their disease happen to them (though my wide eyes and open mouth might tell another tale).

I've lost control of the conversation and spend the next fifteen minutes listening to complaints about pain, uncaring caregivers, the unreliability of Wheel-Trans, the hopelessness of life—each person one-upping the next person's misery. I have nothing but contempt for everyone in the room, a fact that will haunt Future Me, and eventually fill me with grace and compassion (almost) any time I hear a newbie dis the disableds. There is no one-size-fits-all approach to managing MS. The needs of the young and newly diagnosed are as critical as the needs of those with advanced illness, but those needs are fundamentally different. It's not always a good idea to throw us all together in the same room, but where else was I supposed to go?

Just below the surface of my simmering hostility is fear. It's the first time I've been in a room full of people with MS, and coming face to face with what could happen to me is traumatizing. When the blind guy mentions that he likes his neurologist, who happens to be Dr. Poker Face, never mind that Dr. Poker Face didn't prevent him from going blind, I decide, *That's it. I'm out.* I blame nausea from yesterday's injection and get ready to bail out early, because even in my panicked state of mind, I have enough sense not to cop to my revulsion. I promise myself I won't end up like these people.

Before I can leave, a woman about my age enters with her mother. We lock eyes.

"Hi, I'm Sherry," she says, "like the drink."

I sit my ass down, and after the meeting, Sherry and I exchange numbers. Like me, she didn't get much out of the meeting. We decide to start our own support group instead. We can have it in my apartment. There will be Sherry and also wine. Lots of it. Through word of mouth, we discover Darcy, a young woman our age who's had MS for a couple of years. We're excited when she seems interested in joining our Whine Club.

Even more exciting for me is the realization that I already know Darcy, or at least I knew her. It feels like an incredible coincidence, like the universe or Nora Ephron have contrived to reconnect us. We first met in a seventh-grade portable full of French immersion overachievers, but we didn't exactly run in the same circles. For one thing, I didn't run, even before I had any medical reason not to. Darcy had been sporty, popular and cool. I sang Bette's Midler's "Wind Beneath My Wings" at our grade eight graduation and played flute in the band. Lizzo was still a toddler, so the flute wasn't even cool-adjacent back then. I'd chosen it only because piccolo wasn't an option. I was actively anti-athletic and there was no way I was voluntarily making my backpack heavier than necessary. Back then Darcy and I had nothing in common.

We spend the first half-hour of Whine Club on gossip and getting reacquainted. Sherry is single and looking for a career change. Darcy tells us she married her high-school sweetheart. I ask if she's still tight with my seventh-grade crush, Robbie, and she tells me he goes by Rob now, and also he's gay.

We spend the next two hours commiserating over the invisible nature of our symptoms and the frustration of being misunderstood or even, at times, doubted. We are the same age, we're on the same drug and Darcy and I even have the same doctor. With the exception of my vision loss, Sherry's vertigo and Darcy's determination to get pregnant, we have enough in common that we can finish each other's sentences.

I have found my MS friends.

7 / Needle Night

IT'S NEEDLE NIGHT. Half an hour before go-time, I take a pre-filled syringe out of the blue plastic box in my fridge so that the disease-modifying poison can reach room temperature and maybe hurt a little less. Sometimes I forget this step and have to tuck the syringe under my armpit to speed up the process. I lay my supplies out on my bed: a sharps container, alcohol wipes, a towel, an icepack. I keep my auto-injector in the cheap pencil case–type bag it came in. It's the same blue as the box in my fridge, branded with the pharma logo.

"Shit," I say out loud, realizing I forgot the two extra-strength Tylenol that will hopefully take the edge off my needle-night fever. I want to get this over with, but I can't risk getting chills. I down the pills and decide my injection can wait another twenty minutes.

When it's time, I unplug my phone from the jack in the wall. My needle-night ritual is still stressful and scary for me. I need focus and calm; I can't risk being interrupted at a crucial moment. A ringing land line just as I'm about to drive a syringe into my thigh might throw me off like a golfer who hooks his swing when someone coughs.

I consult my drug diary to see which spots are available to me. I have to rotate my injection sites to avoid things like tissue damage and malabsorption. I've been abusing my legs, because it takes contortionist skills to stab myself in the fleshy backs of my arms, and I'm still too grossed out by the thought of injecting my stomach. In truth, I don't really need the book. My body provides a road map of where I've been, with lemon-sized welts and fading bruises in various degrees of freshness marking my flesh.

I prep the auto-injector—a plastic device designed to conceal the needle and make it psychologically easier to self-inject. I swab a reachable section of my ass with an alcohol wipe, then place the plastic tube against my gluteus medius and push the auto-injector's plastic button.

BANG. It's not over yet. I hold the device in place for several seconds while the needle empties. Removing it too early means a hundred dollars' worth of medicine could settle uselessly on my skin. Some days I'm more of a bleeder than others (hence the towel), and it takes quick work to get the used needle out of the way and into the sharps container so that I can put pressure on the site and staunch the bleeding. Finally, I flop back down on my bed, hold the ice to my ass and wait for the flu-like side effects to kick in, relieved to know that I won't have to shoot up again for two more days.

I don't know it yet, but I'm laying the groundwork that will toughen me up. I will never enjoy my thrice-weekly stabbings, but I will get the hang of the routine. Eventually, I won't have to turn off my phone. In fact, I won't even have to put you on hold. I'll be able to shoot up mid-conversation. I'll even be able to take this show on the road and shoot up when it's convenient, whether I'm at a friend's house, a wedding or in an airport bathroom. It's amazing what I will get used to.

In the meantime, there's a knock on my door. I'm not expecting company, which means it must be my friend Sam. Sam lives in Halifax, but whenever he happens to be in town, he shows up unannounced, like a psycho. He has a phone; he just refuses to use it.

"Get your coat. We're going out."

"I can't. I just shot up. I'm about to get the flu."

"Bring the Tylenol. You'll be fine," he insists. If anyone else said this to me, I would be outraged. Sam is the only one of my peers (so far) who has sick-person street cred. We've been close since high school, when we both sang in the Hamilton Children's Choir (HCC).

Sam has a rare and serious congenital multiple-syllabic liver disease. He just calls it Liver Styles. Growing up we never talked about Sam's life-threatening illness. Well, I never talked to Sam about it. The three girls and I that made up the seven members of our tight-knit choir friend group routinely talked about Sam's condition in the way that teenage girls talk about everything: romanticizing the tragedy, filling in the blanks, jumping to conclusions.

"Where are we even going?" I sigh, and Sam can tell he's won.

"Guelph."

"Fucking Guelph? Are you insane? Why?"

"You just have to sit—you don't have to do anything. I promise you'll be okay."

"You're a maniac," I say, as I grab my denim jacket and follow him out the door.

It takes an hour to get to the university town where Sam went to school. Eventually we end up at a club where Sam knows the DJ from the days when, just a few years ago, Sam himself was known as DJ Dr. Strangeliver.

Sam rolls the dice on his strange liver and orders a beer while I respect my pending fever and unpredictable bladder and stick to tiny sips of ginger ale. We hang out for a while, then stop at a hot dog vendor on our way back to the car. It's almost midnight, an hour that never used to feel late but now seems utterly unfamiliar. The street is busy with people flooding in and out of bars, two guys are fighting and there's a girl across the street puking into a garbage can. It's very exciting.

When Sam's buddy, the DJ, comes running out after us, trying to convince us to come to an afterparty, Sam declines without making it feel like I'm the reason.

I have an amazing night. I'm a bit achy, I almost certainly have a low-grade fever, but I barely notice because I'm distracted—I'm having fun. It's good to be out, to be doing something normal. This evening feels like a turning point.

Maybe I don't have to be so precious with myself after all.

8 / Last Meal

ANOTHER ATTACK FOLLOWED BY another round of steroids, and plenty of comfort food, trick me into gaining twenty pounds over the next few months. I choose not to notice. My lingering symptoms remind me that "remission" isn't exactly *le mot juste* to describe the periods between relapses. If a relapse is an MS ten, the time between isn't zero—it's more like a fluctuating three to five. Still, I'm feeling better than I ever thought possible, considering my diagnosis. I have moments of wigging out but I'm no longer experiencing daily meltdowns.

I haven't had any singing lessons and I don't know how long this intermission will last, but for now it feels good not to have the pressure to practise or improve from week to week. I'm not dragging myself to Toronto every Saturday, and I don't have to blame lack of ambition or talent. I can blame MS.

Things are weird again with The Bartender. Just when I think we're getting serious, I remember that I've never even been inside his house—the one he still lives in with his parents, which is its own thing. I don't expect to be invited for any sleepovers, but summer's almost over, and they have a pool. A pool feels like a major girlfriend perk that I am being denied. It's more than that, though. The Bartender isn't spending as much time at my place lately, and I wonder if this is all too much. "This" meaning me. Meaning MS. I wonder if he's just biding his time, afraid of what happens to his good-guy reputation if he breaks up with the sick girl.

Things are just as weird at work. There's no way anyone thinks of me as an up-and-comer anymore. I feel more like I'm being tolerated than appreciated. I'm working reduced hours, which means adjusting to a reduced income. I have to fill out miles of paperwork to validate everything I can or can't do. The unspoken (but whispered-behind-my-back) rule seems to be that if you need to tap into your disability benefits (you know, the ones you pay into in case you get a devastating illness), you're only allowed to either be at work or be doing sick-person shit. Suddenly it's everybody's business how I spend my days. The law says I still get vacation time, and, in fact, I'm about to get on a plane for a trip to Italy and France. Big Boss tells me to let HR know—he's not sure people on disability are allowed to leave the country. (Fact check: we are.) I can feel the Disability Police breathing down my neck.

My family doctor (I have one now) has made the questionable decision to give me fifty milligrams a day of prednisone to manage my stamina and fatigue while I'm away. I love this plan, so I don't ask questions, but I have a feeling Dr. Poker Face would object. I tell myself it's just a little baby dose. And although that might sound like addict talk, fifty milligrams is nothing compared to the gram a day I got with my first relapse back in January (and then again when I relapsed in May). Still, it's a significant amount of steroids that will, if nothing else, give me cheese-and-pasta-eating superpowers. I'm about to gain eight more pounds on foreign land.

The Bartender is coming with me, and maybe this trip will make or break us. The Italian leg of our adventure will feature my Boston bestie, Mike, and his of-the-moment girlfriend, an actress, I think. I'm as excited to see Mike as I am to discover Italy.

Mike has had my back since four hours before we met, when we were first-year students at McGill University. I was a late admission, having ditched the Sorbonne at the last minute to follow my then-boyfriend, The Very Tall One (TVTO), to Montreal. I arrived in the middle of frosh week with nowhere to live, so I planned to crash with TVTO and his new roommates for a couple of nights while I searched for my own apartment. Shortly after I'd dropped off my bags, TVTO left his apartment for the day and inadvertently (I'm giving him the benefit of the doubt) locked me out of his room, where I had just put all my stuff. Including my shoes. This was one of many relationship red flags, but that's a story for another book. I had an appointment to see an apartment of my own, and out of desperation, I took the only shoes in the hall closet: a stranger's pair of men's sneakers four sizes too big.

That my new landlord trusted my ability to pay rent when I was clearly stumbling around in someone else's shoes is a hint at how crappy this apartment was.

When I got back to TVTO's place, my boyfriend and his roommates were in the living room. A guy with messy hair and glasses who was playing guitar jumped to his feet. "Hi! I'm Mike," he said, sticking out his hand and flashing the warmest smile. I was still wearing his shoes. I thought he'd be pissed, or at least creeped out, but Mike turned out to be the kind of guy who would have let me keep those shoes. We've been tight ever since.

AIR TRAVEL WITH a carry-on full of pre-filled syringes is surprisingly a non-issue. Score one for my first disease-related travel concern as I try not to think about my unmet obligation to keep said medication refrigerated. The Bartender and I arrive in Rome, weary from the red-eye but excited. We manage to rent Italy's only car with automatic transmission and make a staggering number of hairpin turns on the beautiful—if nerve-racking—drive to the private villa Mike's parents have rented for the week.

Before we're even out of the car, the Beck family is in the driveway to greet us. The property is stunning. We are surrounded by rolling mountains, cypress trees and olive groves. There's a massive pool and an outdoor pizza oven. Mike gives me the best hug while his dad, Tom, instructs Sue to go and get the prosecco. "Ard is here!" Happy Hour has begun. Mike's parents have always been welcoming to me, but letting us crash their luxury vacay is next-level. I don't think about it too much, but I know I'm here because of MS.

The Becks are cultured, educated, unassuming New England types. Whenever Tom and Sue visited Mike at McGill, they insisted on taking his best friends out for an extravagant dinner—a baller move to a handful of struggling students.

Tom and Sue are invigorated by the company of young people. Tom especially is the kind of parent who likes to party with the next generation, but the evenings they facilitate always have a *salon*-quality feel. We talk about politics, arts and ideas as we drink their good wine. Despite their privilege, there's nothing flashy about the Becks. They are loud. Their sartorial statements make them easily identifiable as American. More than once this week Mike will wear a faded Wonder Bread T-shirt, without irony.

Mike's eyes water when he sees that my walking is so much stronger than the last time we were together, when he flew in to see me shortly after I'd been diagnosed. It takes him a day or two to stop asking if I'm okay. Mike starts to accept that I'm not so fragile, but The Bartender never stops trying to anticipate my needs. To everyone's surprise, including my own, I don't need much help. Italy in August is hotter than the surface of the sun, but somehow (steroid abuse?) I'm able to keep up. I have one little fall and decorate my knee with an impressive scab in Subiaco, and my poor vision makes Michelangelo's ceiling of the Sistine Chapel a bit of a letdown, but MS doesn't ruin *la dolce vita* for me.

We spend the week laughing, eating and drinking all day against a rotating backdrop of cathedrals, palaces and landmarks we recognize from books and movies. At the end of the day, we come back to the villa for late-night swims and midnight pizzas. And the next day we get up and do it all over again. I like The Actress, but I don't bother getting too invested. I can tell Mike's already got one foot out the door. But The Bartender and Mike have instant chemistry and I realize this matters to me. I don't yet know if The Bartender is permanent, but Mike is, and his opinion counts.

It's an emotional day when we leave the Becks for France. Mike and I promise to make plans to see each other, in his country or mine, sometime soon. The Bartender and The Actress beg to be included. Italy has deepened our bond the way shared experiences do.

In Paris, I make sure to keep a steady supply of francs for *la dame pipi*. It's a bit of a panic negotiating my jeans whenever I'm forced to use one of the hole-in-the-ground squatty potties that qualifies as a bathroom in this country, but I manage to avoid suffering any international incidents. I sit out the thirteen-hundred-step climb to Quasimodo's bell while The Bartender makes the trek without me, and even though this is one of my favourite things to do in Paris, I don't feel too sorry for myself. Someone is playing Notre-Dame's famous pipe organ, *and OMG I'm in Paris.*

Nobody says anything about my weight until we get to Nancy. I'm excited to show The Bartender the city where I spent a semester studying classical voice when I was a teen. Nancy is the last stop on our trip, and after ten days of pastries and prosecco, there has never been more of me to love. We get off the train from Gare de l'Est and I scan the crowd, anxiously looking for François and Marie-José, the couple I'd lived with as a student.

"*Oh, là, là*," says MJ, not even trying to conceal her disdain. She gives me *la bise* and then holds me at arm's length. Her "*oh, là, là*" is not the sexy North American false translation *oooh la la*. MJ's "*oh, là, là*" is a low and guttural back-of-the-throat assessment that doesn't end with a whistle of appreciation but a slight head shake and a "bof" of disappointment. By contrast, both she and François are impressed by The Bartender's height. When we get to their home, they insist on measuring him against the wall with the faded pencil dashes that marked the growth of their own kids. They are thrilled to declare The Bartender the tallest person to ever cross their threshold. It's true, I have a type.

My surrogate French parents, the Fossanos, are nothing like my actual parents. I was raised on daily "I love you" reminders and a steady diet of "you can be or do anything you want" (as long as you get a scholarship, because we believe in your dreams but we can't bankroll them). But this is France. My French family is not as easily impressed by what I have been led to believe is my genius and my unlimited talent, beauty and potential. Nonetheless, I don't doubt François and MJ's affection. Their love for me has nothing to do with genetic unconditionality. I earned every kind word or compliment chez Fossano and I understand their tough love is cultural, probably even generational.

François's love language is mentorship, and I showed up at his doorstep as a teen eager to learn. Passionate about French culture, he introduced me to Molière, and Baudelaire, Flaubert and Berlioz. My parents don't know anything about music, and to their ears, every "Ave Maria" I sing is perfect. But François is an actual musician who saw through my shoddy musicianship and tutored me in *solfège*. He took me to chamber concerts and sent me to see *Lohengrin*. Music played constantly from his vast collection of CDs. François coached my Italian arias without flattery, stopping me frequently when he knew I could do better.

Meanwhile, Marie-José's love language is food. It was in Nancy that I first tasted oysters, escargots, champagne, foie gras and frogs' legs. My mornings would start with croissants and *pain au chocolat* so unbelievably good that the dry grocery-store forgeries of my Canadian upbringing quickly became unacceptable to my evolving palate. Baguettes soon redefined bread and I vowed never to consume the bleached sliced stuff again. For lunch, MJ would serve rabbit stew or quiche lorraine with a bacon that was somehow better than bacon, because it was actually *lardons*. MJ had made it her mission to introduce me to as many of France's three-hundred cheeses as possible, and so, any judgment of my weight gain feels pretty rich coming from the woman who taught me to love food in the first place.

But MJ does not punish me for my North American proclivity to overindulge. In fact, she feeds us butter-based dinners, and waters us with unlimited Beaujolais, throughout our four-day stay. Proud of French cuisine and her ability to execute it, MJ can't help making all of my favourite French dishes while we are in her care.

On our final evening in Nancy we have a three-hour, multi-course, wine-paired meal that ends with a selection of not two or three, but eight cheeses. The Bartender is relieved to have not been served anything resembling blood pudding. When we'd first arrived, I made a joke about how much he loves entrails and offal, but the joke didn't translate and MJ thought I was serious, because to them it's just food and *why would that be funny*? Later that night, The Bartender had tried hard to get me to check the fridge and destroy whatever was in there that might make him gag.

François is thrilled with our presence, claiming he doesn't eat this well normally, that MJ is pulling out all the stops. We're all a little bit drunk, and sensing that the evening, and our stay in France, is coming to its end, I feel grateful when François extends the night, asking Marie-José to bring out a little more baguette because there's still a bit more *fromage* on the board. Later, when he asks for more cheese because now there's a bit more bread, MJ brings what's left of the Ribeaupierre, and tells François to give me dibs because this will be my last taste of cheese, my last bite of baguette. I assume I'm being cut off, and that's fine; I have cheese coming out of my eyes. But we've all had more than our fair share, so it seems kind of rude to single me out.

"*Tiens*," says Marie-José, handing me a bag of *fleur de sel* so heavy I know it will put my already packed suitcase over the weight limit. I'm confused. "*Cadeaux*," she continues, as she drops a manual on the table in front of me that's even heavier than the salt. The book is called *L'Alimentation ou la troisième médecine*, and she explains to me that a doctor or researcher or some science dude has proven that certain illnesses, including MS, can be cured with diet.

Part of me, a big part of me, wants easy answers for how to manage my MS, although what the book proposes isn't exactly easy. *L'Alimentation* is a collection of bossy directives to basically stop eating everything I've ever eaten (celery sticks with Cheez Whiz, and bootleg Hamburger Helper) and learn how to use food as medicine. MS has eroded my sense of control, but MJ has offered me a tempting way out. Her clever plan to introduce a massively restrictive diet at the end of a fortnight—and, let's face it, a half year—of complete indulgence, when I'm so full and fat there's literally nothing left to tempt me, makes the whole idea easier to swallow. I don't even question the intervention vibes. I'm not yet wary of people offering me miracle cures and unsolicited advice, so I take this tome in the spirit with which it is intended and embrace the new unprocessed, dairy- and gluten-free, mostly raw lifestyle prescribed by my new bible. I'm so enamoured by *la troisième médecine* that I don't bother wondering what the first two medicines are. (Actual medicine, probably. And then what? Astrology? Reiki? I don't know.)

Europe has been good for my soul. I come back to Canada with a renewed sense of optimism. I discover flaxseed, rice pasta, kale and quinoa like I am the Christopher Columbus of health food. I wean myself off of cream and sugar until I'm convinced I enjoy black coffee. Nobody wants to have me over for dinner because there are too many rules.

The Bartender seems different too, in a good way. I don't know what goes on in his head—he's not a talker—but whatever this disease does to give him pause, he always has an arm ready to steady me, and a sturdy shoulder to lean on. He's always looking out for me. Whatever distance was happening between us in the weeks leading up to this trip seems to have narrowed. Our adventure ends with a "what's next?" energy and I'm feeling pumped to find out.

I'm ready to make changes, ready to kick some ass again. I ditch the steroids. I drop all the weight (and then some) by Christmas. I'm working out, eating my greens, doing all the right things to be a model patient.

With the exception of Dr. Poker Face, who uncharacteristically has an ominous reaction when I skip into his office declaring myself basically cured, everyone compliments me for how I'm fighting this disease and winning. My MS is stable and I'm taking all the credit. I have smugly solved MS.

Of course, the flip side of giving yourself props for doing well with this disease, for believing you control the outcome, is what happens when you have another attack. If fighting is all it takes to beat MS, who's the loser when there's another relapse?

9 / Drug Problem

I'M FALLING OVER like one of those fainting goats. I can't focus on work. I'm exhausted all the time, and not because I've been doing stuff. Everything happens for a reason, and in this case the reason is brain damage.

Elbows on my desk, I rest my hands at my temples like blinders, trying to fake a deep engagement with whatever's on my computer screen when really I'm just trying to hide the fact that my eyes are closed. I'm begging my body to wake the fuck up, but it refuses to comply. I decide to give caffeine a shot instead.

On my way to the office cafeteria, someone asks if I need help. For a second I'm confused. *Do I look lost?* Then I realize I've been dragging my hand along the wall as I walk. I must be off-balance. I didn't even know I was doing it.

I manage to make it back to my desk without spilling my Americano, but I eye it suspiciously, knowing a full bladder might make the car ride home dicey, especially if there's traffic. Lately I've been chewing chocolate-covered espresso beans to mitigate the complication of how to consume caffeine without water, but I'm all out.

I still don't know how to tell if I'm having an attack or if this is what I should expect from MS. I call the clinic for advice and tell my nurse, Maryanna, in a bit of a panic, that I think my MS is getting worse.

"There are good days and bad. Pace yourself. Get enough rest." She sounds rehearsed, like she's been trained to slow her rate of speech and drop her tone of voice to temper hysterical outbursts, but I'm not in the mood to be calmed down.

"I'm hardly doing anything. I can barely keep my eyes open."

"Well, it is what it is," she says with a sigh, like she's the one who gets to be exasperated. She may as well have said, *This is boring. I don't care.*

When Maryanna finally books me an appointment with Dr. Poker Face, he looks alarmed by my weakness. I'm grateful to be taken seriously, but "alarmed" is an off-brand reaction for my unflappable physician. I'm more anxious than ever now. He tells me it's unusual to have so many attacks in the couple of years since my diagnosis. He orders blood work and sends me straight to the hospital to start another five-day course of steroids. When Maryanna meets me in the infusion room, I feel vindicated. I told you I was sick.

Two weeks later my walking is improving, and once again I've never felt more grateful for anything, ever. It's the second-best feeling in the world. (The first best feeling is taking basic functioning for granted.) The emotional extremes of despair and relief are dizzying and my baseline is already kind of off-balance. I need off this roller coaster.

My blood tests reveal that I have developed a clinically significant number of neutralizing antibodies to my MS medication. That's 134 to be precise, when an acceptable number by the design of this test would have been fewer than twenty. *FML*. Neutralizing antibodies mean that, for who knows how long, the injections I've been enduring have been useless. Dr. Poker Face tells me to take what's left of my stash out of the fridge and return it to the pharmacy.

I have "failed" on this drug, though it feels a lot like this drug has failed *me*. This medication was supposed to reduce my relapses by one-third, but nobody could tell me how many relapses to expect. I assumed that if I hadn't been on the drug, I would have been having even more attacks. How was I supposed to know? How is anyone?

Now I need a month-long medically mandated wash-out period—a detox before I can start a new drug, and it's making me uneasy. I feel vulnerable and exposed, like I've gone on vacation and left my apartment unlocked. I have no chill about being on no medication.

The new drug Dr. Poker Face prescribes makes similar claims of reducing relapses by a lousy third. I don't like the numbers. One-third of a figure no one can provide feels like made-up bullshit math. There has to be something better than this. (*Says who?*)

I ask Dr. Poker Face about the stem cell trial I've been hearing about, but he shuts down the conversation, telling me the risks are too high. Dr. Poker Face can't get past the 5 percent mortality rate—even if I can. So, I'm stuck on this janky roller coaster waiting for the next downward spiral until something better comes along.

10 / Capital-A Anxiety

SIX MONTHS LATER, I hate MS so much. Handling it gracefully is exhausting. Except apparently I'm not handling it gracefully. When I tell Dr. Poker Face how much I'm wigging out, he tells me to talk to my family doctor about antidepressants.

I take an unreasonable amount of offence to this suggestion. It makes sense to me that my mood would improve if my symptoms did—and so maybe we should start with the stem cell transplant—but that option's not on the table.

I don't think I'm depressed. I think I'm having the appropriate reaction to living with the constant threat that MS poses to my job, my benefits, my relationships, my vision, my hearing, my ability to walk, all while constantly looking for the nearest bathroom.

Depression feels like a dirty word because if I'm depressed I have failed at having MS. A positive attitude was supposed to save me. Rule Number One of being sick forever: *Keep your chin up. Grin and bear it.* I worry I've failed the people around me, the co-conspirators in the palatable "handling it like a boss" narrative I've assumed.

I have no interest in having a mental health convo with my family doctor, a guy who is good for the occasional round of antibiotics or refill on my EpiPen—but when I needed a pap test, he handed me a Ziploc bag and a Q-tip the length of my arm and told me to leave the sample at the front desk. Once, when I complained of back pain, he told me I probably hurt myself vacuuming. (A statement as misogynistic as it is impossible. I don't even own a vacuum.) And anyway, adding another medication to my daily cocktail might interfere with my ability to consume actual cocktails. No thanks. I reluctantly decide to look into therapy instead.

It takes serious life skills to live with MS, and I resent that I have to spend bus fare and my limited energy cultivating those skills just to be able to function. This is my first experience with professional counselling and I'm skeptical. I don't need someone else to tell me I'm turning into my mother.

My appointment with the MS clinic social worker is at Mac, the hospital where I was diagnosed. So, already a location haunted by trauma. I get lost trying to find the counsellor's office and the extra steps I'm forced to walk are so fatiguing that I feel more demoralized than usual by the time I finally arrive. I feel lied to about the nature of therapy when I discover that there is no Victorian fainting couch for me to recline on while I sort out my existential woes in a cramped institutional space. There are only hard hospital chairs, fidget toys and the low buzz of fluorescent lights.

The social worker has short, spiky, bleached hair and New Age hippie vibes. The books on her shelf tell me she's into meditation. She's probably vegan. I think I see a dream catcher, and I already hate it here. Fortunately, Val uses the F-word within the first few minutes of our appointment and this makes me open to trusting her.

Before we can get into "what's wrong with me," Val lays out the rules. If I tell her I'm going to kill myself, she can't let me leave. Fair enough. I assure her that I might be pissy but I'm not suicidal. I'm not even depressed! But she's not done with her caveats. If I tell her I'm going to kill someone *under the age of sixteen*, she will have to call the cops. That can't be right. I must have misunderstood. I don't ask for clarification, though. I don't want it to sound like I'm looking for loopholes, or that I want to murder Maryanna, who is definitely on the other side of sixteen.

Before I think I've said anything meaningful, Val is already taking notes on a big yellow notepad. How many people will have access to these notes? A stranger's interpretation of my psyche. I'm pretty sure Dr. Poker Face would rather clean toilets than take a peek at my inner thoughts, but what about Maryanna? What about my asshole insurance company?

Val explains depression as mourning the past, and anxiety as fear of the future, and now I have a name for what I'm feeling. Capital-*A* Anxiety. Val agrees that my anxiety is the logical response to some seriously stressful circumstances.

I don't enjoy the experience of anxiety, but I'm not convinced I should try to conquer it either. Anxiety is useful. Anxiety is what got me the appointment that led to the steroids, that led to finding out about those neutral fucking antibodies. Anxiety motivates me to take painful-side-effect-y medication. Getting over anxiety feels like I would be letting my guard down, and letting my guard down feels like an open invitation to MS.

There's nothing Val or anyone can do about what I believe is the real problem: that I have MS. The best she can do is to make me okay with it and I'm not convinced that being okay with having MS is a healthy goal. I think back to an event I attended when I was first diagnosed—a "Welcome to MS" information night when Mac's top neuro talked to patients about treatments and research. When he said that in all of his years of treating MS the patients who did the best were the ones who accepted their diagnosis, I was outraged. I thought he was a quack. What kind of doctor tells you to kick back and accept it? My intention is to fight this disease with everything I've got, and to me that means being on high alert.

Of course, the cost of my vigilance is steep and unsustainable. Every day, I wake up worrying about my next relapse, but crying and freaking out don't seem to be staving off attacks. I don't know how to *not* be scared of what is unquestionably scary. Although most of my moods are future-based daymares, I can't deny that I miss the old *me*. I miss all of the *me*s I could have been if MS hadn't entered the picture. Maybe I *am* depressed. I book a follow-up appointment and get on the bus to go home.

11 / Enough

MY PARENTS HAVE CANCELLED Easter dinner. Holidays are a non-negotiable big deal in my family and so it feels strange to be sitting this one out, but my dad has been unwell and there's no way Norma can pull off a turkey dinner on her own. My siblings and I are left to fend for ourselves, but none of us is at a life stage where it would even occur to us to host a holiday shindig. My younger sister, Corinne, lives in somebody's basement and my little brother, James, still lives at home. I don't own a dining room table (or even a dining room), let alone the flatware to accommodate five people. The only real food I know how to make anyway is one salmon fillet at a time on my tiny George Foreman grill.

No problem. I *do* know how to make my own Easter basket (high-end chocolate from Walker's and six or seven mini-bar-sized bottles of whatever's on sale at the liquor store checkout). As for dinner, I have a boyfriend, and I've been hearing all about The Bartender's complicated, symbol-heavy Ukrainian Easter traditions for a couple of years now. I would never actively choose cabbage and hard-boiled eggs over stuffing and mashed potatoes, but this is an exceptional situation. Although I still haven't been to The Bartender's parents' house for dinner (or for anything else, for that matter), I'm confident he's not going to abandon me on Easter. I mean, I'm mostly confident. Confident-ish. For at least a week, I've been feigning interest in wanting to see for myself just how strong you have to make homemade horseradish to invoke the passion of Christ, but every time I reference the Resurrection, The Bartender finds something else to talk about.

By the time Good Friday rolls around, I figure my chez Bartender invitation must have gotten lost in the mail. FOMO is taking a back seat to my growing anxiety that our relationship can't possibly be as serious as I'd thought. Not being asked to dinner on a major holiday when I've been recently, if temporarily, orphaned is the kind of move that feels like a classic passive-aggressive breakup. I assume The Bartender doesn't want to do the dirty work of telling me he doesn't see this relationship going anywhere, and shutting me out of his family is the action that speaks a thousand douchey words. I decide to confront him. If this relationship is on the rocks, I'm gonna make him say it.

I call him, expecting to hear some not-ready-to-commit bullshit. I am not remotely prepared for the message I eventually extract. He doesn't want to break up, but I can't come for dinner either. He's refusing to tell me why. He wants me to "trust him" and to "let it go." At this point, I feel compelled to reintroduce myself.

"Hi, I'm Ardra. Nice to meet you. Letting things go is not a part of my brand."

And now he's mad at me. "Fine," he says, full of frustration. "What's the ONE THING you have that no one else does?"

I am dumbfounded. And just as frustrated. I literally say, "RED HAIR?" because to me, my hair is the most obvious thing that makes me stand out. But my dye job has nothing to do with my dismissal and I'm out of guesses. I press on. I need him to spell it out for me, and I'm not trying to be an asshole about it. I legitimately can't fathom what the problem could be.

It's not you, he tells me. Not exactly. It's my MS.

The Bartender hasn't told me that his dad can't handle my medical status, because The Bartender has been trying to protect me. Now he's pissed because I made him say this heinous thing out loud. At first I don't understand: Parents are my jam. In high school I was the girl you brought home if you wanted to impress Mom and Dad. A straight-A student, clever and charming, I was a modern-day, Catholic school, female version of Eddie Haskell. The Bartender's parents don't even know me. I'm sure that if they just spent five minutes with me, they'd see how lucky their son is to be dating me. The Bartender assures me that his mom is on my side (our side?), but that she doesn't have a voice. This family is an old-school patriarchy, where whatever Papa Bartender says goes. And Papa Bartender's objection to my MS is so strong that I'm not even welcome in their house. Like I'm fucking contagious.

I'm stunned. The Bartender tells me this is a family matter and that he will deal with it, which only makes me feel more excluded. I know I'm about to start crying hard. I get off the phone and immediately call my parents. Jim and Norma are a guaranteed bag of cocaine for my injured ego, and they say all the right things about how I am a prize and that Papa Bartender is a complete fucking fuck. (I'm paraphrasing, but this is for sure what they mean.)

I'm uncertain of how my call with The Bartender ended. As gutted as I'm feeling, he's struggling too. I knew there had been something going on between The Bartender and his dad for the past few months, I just didn't know it was about me. I flash back to New Years, when The Bartender and I flew to Boston to see Mike. I had wrangled my dad into driving us to the airport. When we picked The Bartender up at his house, I didn't even have a chance to get out of the car before he was rushing toward the driveway with his luggage. As we pulled away in my dad's minivan, Papa Bartender stood in the doorway, unsmiling, his mouth like a hyphen and his arms crossed over his barrel-chested, former-football-player physique. At the time, I'd clocked this as an anti-social *bon voyage*. Now I realize it was open hostility.

Over the next few months, I tell the story of the epic Easter dis to anyone who will listen. I naively have an expectation that this fundamentally misguided judgment of me will be met with the appropriate degree of outrage and incredulity. I am defensive and indignant. I point out that I don't need anyone to look after me. My MS is under control and I expect it to stay that way, even though I know this shouldn't matter. But I am injured all over again when half of everyone I talk to takes Papa Bartender's side. *He just wants what's best for his son* is a refrain I hear enough times to finally stop telling the story. Nothing feels more pathetic, more demoralizing, than trying to convince someone else of my worth. The number of people who can look me in the eye and reinforce the notion that I might wreck someone's life is a gut-punch that I learn to stop inviting.

Until now, the idea that MS makes me "not good enough" has been mostly theoretical—my impression of what people might be thinking, supported by a mental catalogue of micro-aggressions that remind me I'm different. The insidious silent pressure to continuously quantify what I bring to the table was a struggle that, until this incident, I could tell myself was self-imposed, a paranoid overreaction.

But I can't convince anyone of my worth. I am shaken but I stand my ground. I will not accept something as truth just because it's someone else's truth. I will not let Papa Bartender's beliefs about me change what I believe about myself. In fact, I will prepare myself a big plate of Ukrainian kielbasa, because I looked it up, and for some reason, according to the Ukrainians, kielbasa symbolizes God's favour and I'm pretty sure God's on my side on this one.

Papa Bartender may have won Easter dinner, but I already know, and maybe he knows too, that if he doesn't back down, he may lose his son. This standoff has been festering for months. If The Bartender was going to cave to his father's demands, surely he would have done so by now. And anyway, any man worth having doesn't choose his father over the woman he loves.

I tell myself again and again that the people who can't see my worth don't make me worthless. I learn to accept that there will always be those who can't imagine having a partner with MS, a partner like me, and that's fine. It doesn't make me "less-than." It makes them "not enough."

12 / Love Triumphs

SIXTEEN MONTHS LATER, The Bartender and I are at the top of the Arc de triomphe, gazing down the Champs-Élysées, watching the sun set behind the Eiffel Tower. Jet-lagged and drunk on the romance of Paris, I think about how The Bartender has grown into the partner I always dreamt of. Curious and open to new experiences, he wants to travel to every continent and swim in all five oceans. He finally seems ready to break free of the insular world he was raised in.

This is a guy who's solid and reliable, calm in a storm. He can roll with any crowd. He doesn't care about camping, and he never pressures me to watch sports. We laugh at the same things, and our jokes land perfectly in each other's ears. He sees me and backs my big ideas, even when my pie-in-the-sky proposals give him a pragmatic amount of concern. When I'm with him, I am inspired to be the best version of myself. He's someone I trust to keep me safe, to catch me when I fall.

As I turn my gaze from the Eiffel Tower, I see that The Bartender has dropped to his knee, a small navy blue box in his palm. I don't squeal or cry when I see the ring. I don't have an outsized reaction when he asks me to marry him. I just say yes because it feels so obvious. It just feels right. Like we are supposed to be. Love triumphs.

13 / Forced Ranking

I'M THE LAST ONE to arrive at the middle-management meeting and it's standing room only.

"I'll be right back. I'm just gonna grab a chair." This should be an empty offer. There are only three chairs in Big Boss's office and not much room for a fourth, considering that the whole supervisory team is in here. I don't expect Big Boss himself to relinquish the big leather throne he's perched on behind the desk that separates him from his lowly subjects, but I'm annoyed when Dave and Diana, the two able-bodied seat hoarders, call my bluff. I leave in frustration to get a chair.

Three years after my diagnosis, the initial outpouring of love I'd received from my co-workers has morphed into something more like low-key resentment. The company culture is as cutthroat as ever, and while everyone else is working overtime trying to prove their worth, I'm keeping part-time hours that are topped up by disability benefits. I'm rolling into work when I feel like it. I recently spent a girls' weekend in NYC. I don't look sick. I look twenty-seven. I've got good skin and a great haircut. People find it hard to believe what they can't see. Recently, someone even asked me, "Are they *sure* you have MS?" and it felt like more of an accusation than an inquiry.

At this point, dear reader, your outrage may be directed at me. I mean, how could I jet off to NYC while I was receiving workplace accommodations and benefits? Never mind that it's actually nobody's business how anyone spends their hours when they're not at work. I should have been sick in bed, living my sick and sad life. The rule is that anyone who needs help must be helpless, dependent, pitiful. Poor.

I feel this judgment from my co-workers too. Not all of them, but it takes only one or two raised eyebrows and a snide comment to poison my psyche—to make me come undone. I get defensive. I feel like I have to justify everything, explaining that I want to travel while I still can. I share excruciating details about how MS impacts me in an effort to have my illness taken seriously, as if explaining invisible symptoms ever helped a skeptic understand anything. My justifications only make me doubt myself.

As I struggle to open the door and squeeze a chair into the crowded office, it's a beat too long before someone says, "Oh, do you need help with that?" And anyway, there's a weird hush in the room, like they've just been talking about me.

"We were just wondering if anyone was throwing you a lingerie shower for your wedding," Kate says and everyone laughs. *Wait, is that a snicker?*

"Oh, you don't have to throw me a shower," I answer awkwardly. "I've already had three!" I blurt before thinking about which one of my colleagues might feel pissy about not having been invited. (Mindy, it's definitely Mindy.) But the lingerie question is such an uncomfortably weird thing to suggest in your boss's co-ed office that I feel like I need to fill the air. I'm about to blab on about the wine shower my cousin Laura hosted when Kate jumps back in.

"Oh, no, we weren't offering; we just thought you could use some thongs," she adds, raising an eyebrow and nodding at my ankle-length charcoal-grey knit skirt. My face goes red as I start to understand. Maybe an ass-skimming skirt when you need a bit of bladder protection is a fashion failure on my part, but Kate knows about my issues. Not because she's someone I wanted to confide in, but because I needed her to understand why I couldn't continue to lead two-hour workshops without ad hoc bathroom breaks. Now she's mean-girling me in front of the whole team.

"Let's get started," Big Boss says, saving me from having to reply or burst into angry, embarrassed tears.

The tech bubble is bursting and the organization is downsizing, though nothing official has been said. Morale is bad. Everyone's on edge; there's lots of whispering. The walls of Big Boss's office are covered with a dozen pages of flip-chart paper, each labelled with "twenty," "seventy" or "ten." Our task today is to use Jack Welch's dehumanizing system of identifying the most valuable 20 percent of workers, the average 70 and the "go fuck yourself" 10. The office windows are blacked out so that our staff on the other side can't see what we're up to.

Once we've decided which category someone lands in, we then have to rank each employee within that category and add their names with Magic Markers to the papered walls in order of best to worst. We're looking for weakest links, the 10 percent of people who will be the first to get fired, but not the last.

The room seems divided into the bleeding hearts who don't want to fire any of the single moms or recently widowed and the ruthless who seem capable of seeing the employees as numbers and not as people. Everyone agrees that John is a space cadet, but when one of the other supervisors objects to putting him dead last on the loser list, on the grounds that he is "so nice," Big Boss reminds us that we are not Santa Claus. Dave proposes we get rid of Stella so that she can turn her gambling addiction into a full-time gig. I'm pretty sure the suggestion of what to do about the four women currently on mat leave is illegal. Ranking each person against their co-worker is incredibly subjective, and it feels like gossipy dirty work. The process is bringing out the worst in us.

Although I'm part of the team tasked with deciding the fates of our lowest-level employees, I know there's another room, bigger than this one, that has my name on a chart somewhere too.

Over the past six months or so, Big Boss has been bouncing me around, putting me in different roles, and each one seems a little less accommodating than the last. I can't tell if the goal is to break me or if the company is trying to do me a favour by proving it can't accommodate me, so that I qualify for long-term benefits.

I don't want to stop working, even if I am miserable in this job: there's nowhere else to go, and nobody would hire me given my pre-existing list of limitations. I don't know what happens to my MS without medical insurance, without medication.

My symptoms are invisible but the writing is literally on the wall: I'm getting fired or I'm about to be medically retired.

14 / Home Is Where the Elevator Is

"YOU CAN WEAR HEELS?" Darcy accuses, before she's even out of her car.

"You can drive!" I say from the sidewalk where I've been waiting outside The Bean Bar, the restaurant I suggested for its velvet banquettes, sweet potato fries and proximity to my apartment. MS robbed Darcy of her ability to wear heels, whereas I lost the right to drive on Day One, after I never fully recovered from optic neuritis. I know it's not a contest, but limited transportation options feels like as much of a raw deal as any fashion dilemma.

Darcy and I are meeting for lunch, where we will be surrounded by people who, I assume, are capable of both wearing heels and driving, but Darcy and I never bother comparing ourselves to civilians. We don't lament the health of healthy controls. We keep our envy realistic by restricting our comparisons to others with MS. Anyway, we're not out to make each other feel bad. We're overdue for a catch-up—it's been months since Darcy hosted one of her wine-soaked Friday Girls' Nights, and I've got wedding plans to share.

When Darcy gets out of her car, she pulls a cane out of the back seat. In the three years since we've reconnected, this is the first time I've seen her with a mobility aid, and the effect is jarring.

"I can get by without it," she says, noticing me notice, "but I can't take another asshole yelling at me for parking in the accessible space." The Disability Police are always lurking, eager to publicly shame anyone they suspect might be taking advantage of the system. The presence of a cane means Darcy's more likely to get side-eyed than screamed at by the vigilantes who don't know anything about invisible illness. But her movements are stiff. She's not limping exactly; it's more like her knees don't want to bend. She definitely needs that cane. Suddenly my optic neuritis doesn't seem so bad.

We make our way inside the crowded café, and when the hostess asks where we'd like to sit, we both, at the same time, ask for the booth closest to the bathroom and then start laughing.

"She's pregnant," Darcy tells the hostess. It's a bald-faced lie that nets us the table we asked for. Ordering that cocktail is going to be awkward, but our inside joke reminds us that we are on the same team.

"Tell me everything," Darcy says once we've settled in. I'm happy to blab. I'm not even close to tired of telling the story of how The Bartender proposed in Paris.

"Are you going to change your name?"

"I thought about it"—not really—"but I can't imagine being Mrs. Someone Else."

"I couldn't wait to change my name," Darcy says, smiling at the memory.

"Yeah, but you've got a good one. *Darcy Hewitt* sounds like a news anchor or a romance novelist. The Bartender's last name sounds like how you spell a sneeze."

"Maybe he'll change his name to Shephard."

"Ew," I say. "That's almost as bad. I think we'll go with a brand-new name and call ourselves Shepinetz."

"A 'ship name! Cute!" Darcy says. "Like Brangelina!"

I agree. "Actually, I was hoping to co-opt your next Friday Girls' Night," I continue, eager to talk wedding plans. Friday nights in Darcy's cozy subterranean lair typically involve a collection of her girlfriends, mostly soccer moms eager to trade their kids and husbands for an evening of drinking and gossip, while crafting Christmas cards, scrapbooking or humouring Darcy's latest MLM pyramid scheme. For a few hours a month, I dip my toe in suburbia, and try not to admit how much I like it.

"I'm thinking of making the wedding invitations myself. I want to do a travel theme. The invites could look like antique postcards."

"Love it."

"I'm hoping you can help me with the card design and then we could get the girls to help make them." Darcy's basement is stocked like a craft superstore. Her professional-grade paper cutters alone would make the task a breeze. "It's only about 110 invitations. Maybe 120. I'll bring the wine and snacks. And, anyway, we're due for a Girls Night—"

"Ard," she stops me. "I can't."

"Is this a bad time? The wedding's not until October . . ."

"We put the house on the market."

"What? But you love that house!"

"Well, the house doesn't love me." Darcy looks sad and angry. Heartbroken. "I haven't been near the basement in weeks. There *are* no more Friday Girls' Nights. I can handle one or two stairs, but I can't do a whole flight of stairs. It's impossible."

Darcy has made her nest, filled it with a husband and kid, and lined it with scrapbooking paper. Meanwhile, I'm still a drifter who's never had any real attachment to an address. At twenty-seven, I've already lived in fifteen different places. From houses to apartments to crash pads, in southern Ontario, Quebec and even France, home has never felt like an address to me—home is a state of mind.

In contrast, The Bartender just turned thirty and he's still living in the same mid-century, two-car-garage detached suburban home where his father wins municipal awards every year for his hostas and superior landscaping. The Bartender knows his neighbours, and hasn't had to memorize a new postal code every 1.8 years.

As our wedding date approaches, it's time for The Bartender and I to make a home together. The real question isn't what to call myself, but where The Bartender and I will live.

Choosing our first home together involves considerations beyond my fiancé's deluded fantasies of tending his own garden and my preference for the sound of traffic over the sound of children playing. As a non-driver, city life, access to public transit and walkability scores mean independence to me.

Although autonomy has long been at the top of my dream-home wish list, accessibility isn't something I thought I needed to worry about. But Darcy has two years of MS life experience on me, which makes her a harbinger of things to come. Even in her twenties, Darcy's body is forcing her whole family's eviction. As if that's not bad enough, apparently affordable bungalows are in low supply and high demand. The struggle to find a house that meets her family's needs is an added nightmare I never want to experience.

Maybe it's optimism bias, but at this stage of my life, I don't actually believe MS will ever land me in a wheelchair—that said, the memory of pulling myself up to my second-storey apartment is not something I want to relive. Darcy's ordeal is the reality check I need to make a case to The Bartender for Urban Centre Elevator Life: a housing crisis prevention plan.

"Pros," I say. "Housing in Hamilton is way cheaper than in Burlington." Fiscal prudence is this guy's jam, so I open strong.

"Cons," The Bartender responds. "Hamilton is farther away from work. It would be a longer commute."

"Pros: It's also farther from your parents' house."

"What? You don't want my dad popping in for random visits and unsolicited advice?"

"Pros: Better nightlife, better restaurants. We could get Bronzie's pizza on the reg," I say.

"What about those brownstone townhouses, close to the bottom of the mountain? I've always loved the look of those."

Bingo. I have achieved urban dwelling buy-in. Time for Phase Two. The brownstones are beautiful but they don't solve the problem. "The walk-ups? I love them, but I think we should find an apartment—a condo without any stairs. Just in case."

"What happened to Darcy isn't going to happen to you. Your legs are strong," The Bartender tries to reassure me.

It's true. Lately my legs have been working as one would expect legs to function. I'm on the treadmill almost every day. But still. "I know it's an abundance of caution, but I never want to get sucker-punched by MS again," I say. "I could have another attack, and even if I recover, it would suck to have to deal with stairs even temporarily." Planning for personal disasters is not the kind of wedding planning I've been looking forward to.

"I guess I could put a couple of tomato plants on a balcony."

The Bartender is on board, nodding his head in agreement, but I try to sweeten the deal because I don't want to start this marriage feeling like we're already making sacrifices for me. "We won't have to shovel snow, mow the lawn or lug garbage to the curb—"

"Of course, Sheppy, these are all pros. You don't have to convince me. We'll find a place that works."

If home is a state of mind, the state I'm seeking is sanctuary. In an attempt to outsmart fate, I tell myself that preparation makes worst-case scenarios less likely to happen. Like a dusty fire extinguisher that never gets used, finding a home that doesn't have stairs feels like a symbolic gesture, an offering to the universe so that the universe will leave me alone.

Although Darcy settles for her next home, having been forced to lower her expectations and let go of her own dream-house wish list, TB and I excitedly look for lofts with views and rooftop patios, hoping to find a Frasier Crane–style space, something that has the energy of *Melrose Place* without the murder. Nobody tell the Universe that Urban Centre Elevator Life hardly feels like a sacrifice to us.

That the mere absence of stairs doesn't necessarily make a home accessible is a lesson I won't have to learn for another fifteen years.

15 / Lucky

IT'S THE DAY BEFORE MY WEDDING, or, as The Bartender points out, *our* wedding. Except obviously I'm not marrying a nightclub bartender with a soul patch. I'm an adult and, suddenly, so is he. Although the sketchy facial hair disappeared some time before we were engaged, The (now former) Bartender tended his last bar a week ago. He's leaning into his full-time gig in finance now, and so The Bartender becomes The Banker. It doesn't matter that he doesn't actually work at a bank. The Mutual-Funder is too much of a mouthful. And anyway, I'm not entirely sure what he does. He's the Chandler Bing of our friend group, and so *Banker* feels close enough.

My (our) dream wedding is in Ontario's wine country. It's late October and the fall leaves are at their most magnificent. The 1860s small wooden chapel where we will seal the deal is so lovely that I can't stay mad about the words *Balls Falls* appearing on our invitations. The church is next door to a waterfall (the "falls" in *Balls Falls*), but its most charming feature is the steeple's iron bell, which is attached to a rope near the entrance. My kid cousin Christopher will ring it after the ceremony as The Banker and I make our way out of the church to the overture from Mozart's *Marriage of Figaro*.

Everyone we love is here. Mike has flown in from New York. My maternal grandmother, G, as we call her, is here from Montreal. Even Papa B has come around. Sort of. "If you're happy, I'm happy" is a bare-minimum statement of support. I know because I used the same line at my sister Corinne's first wedding when I couldn't think of anything nicer to say about her confounding choice of (temporary) partner. Whatever. I don't sweat it. He's here, despite his failed attempt to make me sign a pre-nup. A decision he comes to accept because, as he repeatedly reminds both me and my fiancé, spouses have no legal claim on their partner's inheritance. (Like they're the fucking Vanderbilts and not a couple of retired teachers.) Anyway, it's good news for The Banker, who dodges an exceptionally large hat-collection bullet from my side of the family.

At five o'clock, it's already dark when we arrive for the rehearsal. We're barely out of the car when my mom appears out of nowhere, grabs my arm and starts pulling me toward my dad's minivan.

"I have a surprise for you," she sings.

"Can't we do it after? We're going to be late." She has not let go of my arm.

"Trust me, you're gonna want this."

As we approach the van, a petite curvy figure swathed in a scarf the size of a duvet steps out of the shadows and I lose my mind. It's Marie-José. She's been hiding out at my parents' place for the past two days, preparing all my favourite French foods for the post-wedding brunch. After trying to teach Norma how to make a proper tarte Tatin by email, she finally realized it was futile and declared with a heavy accent, "I must come to Canada!" (And yeah, I'm eating cheese again.) François was not able to travel, but composed a four-part chorale for the occasion. I'm overwhelmed with excitement and surprise. I squeal "Oh my god!" eighteen times before I calm down long enough for MJ to hold me at arm's length and issue her assessment. I'm wearing a black turtleneck, knee-high boots and a narrow printed skirt, my own foulard slung casually around my neck. She nods in approval. "*Tu as l'air d'une vraie française.*" It's the highest compliment she can give or that I can receive.

The rehearsal goes well. Naturally. I'm prepared and organized, determined to pull off a perfect day. Of course, there is no rehearsal for what I'm most worried about—that my MS-y bladder and bowel will fail to co-operate. I'm hyper-aware of the bathroom location at every point over the next couple of days. There's no toilet in the one-room church, but there are public washrooms in the park across the street, where there are also definitely spiders. Not ideal. My plan is to limit fluids and food and say a few strongly worded prayers. If Jesus is busy, I'm willing to hear what kind of deal Satan has to offer. I want to keep MS as far away from this day as possible.

The Banker and I are staying in separate rooms at the same B & B, keeping things tradish. Not biblically, of course. It's just that I want the deluxe fairy-tale package. I insist we spend the night and the next day apart to heighten the drama and anticipation of the moment when we meet at the altar. I have stage-managed the shit out of this production and I want it to be flawless. Plus, I need some sleep if I'm gonna function. The plot hole in my plan is that although I fully anticipate that tomorrow will be the best day of my life, I also expect it to be the longest. I already know that, by the end of the night, I will be too tired to consummate this thing—a quintessential wedding experience, from what every movie tells me. The night before our wedding, at just after midnight, I'm still wide awake when I consider that, technically, today is tomorrow. It's our wedding day. I tiptoe downstairs and knock quietly on TB's door. I explain the situation and he is, of course, on board to outsmart MS. Afterward, we give each other a comparatively chaste kiss good night and I sneak back to my room. The next time I see him will be at the church.

I'm late for the ceremony because that's also a tradition, and for good reason. I refuse to arrive before potentially tardy guests, and also a swarm of ladybugs gets caught in my veil and my bridesmaids have to pick them out, one by one. Then we have to go back for my lipstick. This is my day and I will be as late as I want.

It's a cool autumn afternoon, but the sun is shining. My bouquet of sunflowers reminds me of my beloved France. I'm wearing my dream dress—a Jenny Lee dupion silk, off-the-shoulder gown with ruched chiffon sleeves. It's the only dress I tried on, and if I'd had a million dollars, it's still the one I would have chosen. My bridesmaids are in pink, naturally. I walk down the aisle to Hagood Hardy's theme from *Anne of Green Gables* to meet The Banker at the altar. He's wearing an Armani suit and a tie made from the same ivory silk of my dress. We say our vows clearly and confidently, with unbroken eye contact. And then we're married.

We have pictures taken, and while guests head to the vineyard for cocktails and candy apples, The Banker and I make a quick detour back to the B & B. Not to have sex—that's not on the schedule (and I just told you, we already ticked that box). MS doesn't get a day off, and so neither do I: The Banker helps me out of my gown so that I don't get blood on it. I shoot up and a lemon-sized welt appears on my thigh. It feels like a bee sting. I've given myself almost a thousand injections by now. I take it in stride.

The reception is at a vineyard, in a Teutonic-style wooden building. The covered bridge at the entrance sold us on the venue before we'd even seen the interior or tasted the *poulet-en-croûte*. The dining room is filled with fairy lights, buckets of Halloween candy and a hundred people ready to party. I'm ready to party too, now that I finally have the comfort of knowing I'll be close to a bathroom for the next four or five hours. It's time for champagne. MS has so far blessedly behaved, but there's one last hurdle to get through, and it's the speeches.

Sitting through wedding speeches is the price guests pay for access to an open bar, and if you're lucky, pizza at eleven. Wedding speeches are boring at best. More often, they're humiliating (or hilarious in a *schadenfreude* way, depending on how you feel about the bride or groom in question). I'm not worried about embarrassing stories of youthful shenanigans. I will merely roll my eyes if forced to participate in the clichéd bit where the speech-giver has the groom place his palm over the bride's hand so that he can experience one final moment of having the upper hand. What I desperately do not want to hear are speeches that in any way reference my MS.

My mom tells me and everyone who will listen (which is no one) that, according to proper etiquette, brides are not to be congratulated. Grooms may be congratulated, but brides must only be offered best wishes. I don't need to live by antiquated rules. People have been congratulating me since our engagement one year ago, and I'm cool with it. Plus, *best wishes* kind of feels like a polite version of "it's your funeral/ good luck with that asshole" (something we might have said to my sister). What's irking me is how many congratulations are directed at me with a side order of "you're so lucky." People like to tell me that The Banker is one-in-a-million, and the subtext is that it takes a special kind of guy to marry someone like me, someone with MS. "You're so lucky" sounds like the first half of a sentence that ends with "he's marrying you *even though* . . ."

In a pathetic bid for script approval, I had practically begged everyone preparing a speech not to breathe a word about my health. It's not a secret. Everybody in the room knows I have MS. But wedding speeches tend to have a "this is your life" quality, and I don't want the headline to be "Prince Charming Rescues Damsel in Distress." And maybe this is the universe giving me a fairy-tale wedding after all. Because as it turns out, fairy tales are inherently problematic. "Handsome Hero Marries Brave Girl" is not my narrative, even if it's one others want to project. Nobody who has congratulated The Banker has felt compelled to point out anything about his own good fortune. Someone even asked him if my dad has thanked him, like I'm some kind of problem that needs to be solved, and I don't have to blow my brains out (or anyone else's), because The Banker consistently makes me feel like he's the lucky one. I know I can't control what anyone thinks (trust me, I've tried). I just want everyone to say that I'm a lovely bride without making me feel like this wedding is my Make-A-Wish.

My request is granted, mostly. The MS-iest thing that gets said is from a choked-up bridesmaid when she references "how much I've been through." I gag a little, but I don't die. My uncle Bruce toasts my beautiful smile, my beautiful voice and my passionate nature. My new mother-in-law, Jan, who is model tall and just as thin, steals the scene when she changes out of her mother-of-the-groom frock and into the suit her father wore at his wedding in the 1940s. It fits her perfectly. She says, "Ardra is not my daughter-in-law, she is my friend." My dad's speech brings down the house. It's funny and poignant. He does not thank The Banker for taking me off his hands. When the dancing starts, Papa B tells me that he loves me. It's the first tender moment I've ever had with him. He's definitely drunk, but it still feels good. I'm drunk too.

By the end of the night, I'm somehow the last one on the dance floor. The only casualties of an otherwise perfect day are my sore feet and torn and dirty dress. It was a perfect day and not just because I was the centre of attention. My new husband and I were both at the centre of the joy and love and support of a hundred people. There's magic in having your whole posse of people in one room at the same time, rooting for your happiness.

Buzz kills and marriage counsellors caution that it's not the party that matters, but the marriage that comes next that counts. I think that's only half-true. Parties aren't just "nice-to-haves." This party reminded me that I have a team of people with big and small long-term and transient roles to play in my life. Our life. Good people who care if I live or die. As I'm falling asleep mid-sentence, it's a feeling I try to memorize. I want to store it somewhere deep and permanent, treat it like it's a living thing. So that when times are tough, I can remind myself that MS is lonely, but I am not alone. This is why we party.

16 / Things I Did When I Wasn't Watching *Oprah*

I'M TAKING MY VITAMINS, exercising and eating well (mostly). I'm shooting up at the same time every day, rotating my sites—I've even figured out how to inject my arms. I'm showing up for all my appointments, and monitoring my MS.

Hamilton isn't Paris or New York, Montreal or even Toronto, but it *is* a city with galleries, an opera company, a university, a scene. Our fifteen-hundred-square-foot downtown loft is the coolest place I've ever called home. We have a sixth-floor view of the city, two bedrooms (the spare one is for guests, not babies) and windows instead of walls. Our home is hip, modern and fab. The location is perfect. I can walk my non-driving, low-vision self to the gym, the market, the art gallery, the movies, the bars and even the symphony.

My husband and I spend the first few months of married life unpacking, finding the perfect place to put our wedding gifts and fighting over whose books deserve the best spots on the shelves. We fill our apartment with oversized art and learn all about feature walls, under-mount sinks and the unlimited shades of white you can paint your baseboards. When we can't decide if we should put the Christmas tree in the bedroom or the living room, we realize we have room for both and get two. But the very best part of our new life together is the addition of a puppy—a floppy good-natured doodle we decide to name Rihga.

She's like a teddy bear with a heartbeat. Playing house is fun.

After MS and marriage, the next thing I get to know about my grown-up life happens around the same time. At twenty-seven years old, I become medically retired: unemployed due to illness. Officially, vision loss, weakness, fatigue and frequent relapses have become too difficult for my employer to reasonably accommodate. Unofficially, you can add incontinence and anxiety to the list. My office days are over. Fortunately, my bougie drugs will still be covered because I'm on The Banker's policy now.

If there's anything good about worst-case scenarios coming true, it's that you get to stop worrying about the horrible thing that might happen. If you don't die, you deal with it. Solving problems, even big ones, is always more satisfying than worrying about them ahead of time.

I'm processing two new identities, one welcome, one fraught. Who I am without meaningful employment is something I still have to figure out, even if my job never felt like a calling. I have an idea about the kind of wife I want to be—but it has never included motherhood, and I can't just be a housewife. I'm pretty messy, and I'm not that nurturing. I can't sit around watching soap operas all day either. I mean, technically I could, we have cable, but I don't want to. I'm adrift and hoping medical retirement will be the crisi-tunity that helps me figure out what to do with the rest of my life.

I call my cheerleader mom to see if she has any insight into my reinvention. She lists all the experiences I've had that fill her with wonder. Whitewater rafting, swimming with dolphins, the strange things I ate as a student living in France. Is it possible for me to find value in experiences instead of accomplishments? Instead of a paycheque? I almost died whitewater rafting, and I'm not really a dolphin person. Cheese is great but food doesn't feel like the foundation of a personality. I don't know what I want to do—let alone what I'm qualified for—but maybe valuing my experiences will help me figure it out.

I make a list of all the things that bring me joy, while wondering just how much joy is socially acceptable for a twenty-something medical retiree. People like to say (with thinly veiled derision) that it "must be nice" to not have to work. And I guess it is nice, at least for the first few days, maybe even the first few weeks. After all, even the best jobs in the world can feel like a grind from time to time. But there's a big difference between not *having* to work and not being able to. Studies have repeatedly shown that the overwhelming majority of disabled people would prefer to work, that disability benefits can feel like a crappy consolation prize for a future without a career.

Having your financial needs met (by someone else, by your benefits or by some combination of both) does not guarantee a feeling of autonomy. Maintaining a sense of self-worth, purpose and dignity can be tough when you feel useless. Being medically retired is not the same thing as being on an extended vacation.

Unconvinced? Imagine there's some kind of global pandemic that keeps you from working. (Now imagine this happens during a time without Netflix, DoorDash, FaceTime or Zoom.) The Canadian government decides most people need two thousand dollars a month to survive. They don't ask too many questions. Unless you're disabled, of course, in which case you can continue to survive on the monthly $1,387.66 (assuming you receive the maximum allowable benefit at the time) that you most certainly had to go to great lengths to prove you even *merit*. Never mind the extra and often exorbitant expenses of being disabled. Or the constant fear of the reassessments that put your meagre benefits at risk.

People receiving disability benefits are expected to exist without really living, and I hate that I have to justify what is actually nobody's business. But we live in a world where we make other people's business our own, especially when we feel things are unfair.

What's actually not fair is that if I weren't married and had to exist solely on my disability benefits, I'd be living below the poverty line, unable to afford my medication. I don't want to reinforce the "must be nice" narrative, when what's nice for me should be a standard of living that's available to everyone who is forced to make managing their bodies their full-time job.

It's a privilege to have the financial security to prioritize my health, and my good luck depends on my partner continuing to be a decent guy—one I want to stay with and who wants to stay with me. (Statistically, though, this is unlikely. Marriage is already a leap of faith, and a significantly higher-than-average number of MS marriages end in divorce, especially in heterosexual relationships where it's the female partner who has MS.)

Like it or not (definitely not), money is power in a relationship—I can't undo centuries of patriarchy. Knowing how fucked you'd be without your husband can set up a dynamic that I have to make an effort to avoid, regardless of the fact that TB doesn't do anything to reinforce any "kept-wife" feelings my insecurities might tempt me to explore.

My story is far from a worst-case scenario. The stress, stigma and difficulty around accessing benefits is exacerbated in proportion to the number of marginalized identities you intersect with. It's a system that can make you feel like a criminal. Some of us will literally end up in court fighting for the assistance we are owed.

Disabled or otherwise, we exist in a culture that doesn't encourage anyone to rest, let alone do anything pleasurable until we've earned it. I have to regularly reassure myself that I am not the second-class citizen some would have me believe. I can't fix our misguided cultural values, but I can say that for anyone facing this situation, I see you. You are not alone. You don't suck at life. You got a raw deal and you don't deserve an obstructive, uncaring bureaucracy on top of everything else you're managing.

It feels subversive to suggest that, like everyone else, I, too, have a right to joy, to purpose, to figuring out how to participate in the world in a way that makes sense for me and my body. I may be too sick to work full-time, but I'm determined to make the most of my life, and so I put aside my concerns about stereotypes and stigma and get back to my list.

Singing doesn't make the cut because it seems so impossible—when I consider my lost potential, it only brings me regret. I focus instead on my love of languages, art, travel, food, books, spending time with friends and the ever-important necessity of looking after my MS. Then I try to figure out how to experience more of these things in manageable, bite-sized pieces.

Every month, I write down the books I read, how much time I spend exercising and doing physio, who I host or have lunch with. If someone sends me an email thanking me for anything, I copy and paste it in a file I call "Things I Did When I Wasn't Watching *Oprah*." I give myself props for Every. Little. Thing. Cataloguing my activities makes me feel like I'm accomplishing something even if my attempt at beef stroganoff tastes like prison food and the smartest book I read is *The Sisterhood of the Traveling Pants.* My self-esteem bible is the evidence I need to convince myself that I might be sleeping until eleven, but I'm not completely frittering my life away.

Still, I feel the need to be excellent at something, to do something more, something artistic. My existential angst is a luxury that's possible only because my health is more or less under control without the demands of work. Except for my daily injections, the need to budget my energy and my constant search for the nearest bathroom, I don't think about MS too much. "How to not waste my life" starts to take up more and more real estate in my mind.

As I noodle through my dilemma in my social worker Val's office, she encourages me not to look outside of myself for life satisfaction. She uses the word *grandiose* and then immediately retracts it when she sees my back go up. I think back to my high-school drama teacher, who wrote in my yearbook, "Ardra, remember to love the art in yourself, not yourself in the art," and feel as misunderstood now as I did then. Maybe it sounds grandiose to say it out loud—that I still want to do big things with my life. Or maybe my problem doesn't merit as much consideration because in the hierarchy of MS problems, self-actualization seems like an extravagance, like too much to ask for. When Val tries to convince me that of course my life isn't ordinary, in the sense that no one's is, I feel like it's time to wrap this appointment up. I don't think of ambition as something to overcome, but it seems like a pretty inconvenient quality for someone in my position.

My brag sheet evolves and grows every month. My confidence in what I can commit to builds, and eventually I start to think about volunteering. In a world where there are no bad ideas, I briefly consider a position as choir director at the Barton Street Jail, until an opportunity to be in a film documentary on a major network steals my focus. The project features direct descendants of Canadian World War I soldiers and nurses. There will be some element of living like our ancestors did during the war, but without actual gangrene or body lice. I assume. The producers are preferencing applicants with access to primary resources and my mom has recently published *Dear Harry*, a collection of my great-grandfather's war correspondence. The project sounds interesting. Some of it is being shot in England, some in Quebec. I'm not a war re-enactment weirdo, but I was moved when, on tour with the HCC, I sang a Canada Day concert at Vimy Ridge, the battle site where my great-grandfather Harry was killed.

When I receive an invitation to participate, I start thinking about what I'm going to pack and who I'm going to meet. But my invite is rescinded after I fill out the medical questionnaire. The producers don't care that my health is stable; MS is a deal-breaker for them. I am too expensive to insure and I'm pretty certain this is discrimination. I decide to feel more dissed than disappointed. Just because I am well enough to sleep in a trench doesn't mean I want to.

When I get a gig as a volunteer docent at the newly renovated Art Gallery of Hamilton, I've already decided that from now on, new people don't get to know my disease status. The AGH has an important collection of nineteenth-century French Romanticism that I'm especially keen to explore. The gallery itself is a beautiful space, and the more time I spend there, the more I start to feel tethered to a community. I start to recognize myself again—the kick-ass version.

Every grade-five class in the city gets to come to the AGH. For many ten- and eleven-year-olds, it's their first-ever experience at an art gallery and I feel privileged to be the one to introduce them to this world. My debut solo tour is with a group of inner-city kids—all boys. I expect it to be a nightmare, the price I have to pay to do the fun stuff of attending art lectures, researching artists and paintings, having coffee with the other docents. But the boys are keen and attentive. They make intelligent observations. It's invigorating. I check in with my ovaries just to make sure we still don't want kids (we don't), but I concede that kids can be kind of cool to hang out with.

I keep my MS incognito by scheduling tours during the narrow window of my most functioning hours of the day. School groups turn out to be more enjoyable than adult tours because the kids don't feel compelled to contribute pretentious observations. Ten-year-olds don't yet know the word *juxtapose*, and when I need to stop at a bench, I can ask them to sit on the floor while I teach them how to read a painting.

Gallery life is so rewarding that even when I don't win Docent of the Year (though I am nominated), I realize that I don't need to be the best to feel a sense of purpose, to feel filled up. Val will be impressed.

THE MORE I get my shit together, the more I realize how much I miss singing. Auditions are being held for a local Gershwin revue and the theatre is within walking distance from our apartment. The location is so convenient and Gershwin is so singable that prepping an audition doesn't feel overwhelming or like much of an investment. I don't get my hopes up, but when I get a phone call offering me a role, I'm surprised by my own excitement and do a happy dance in the kitchen.

It feels so good to be going to rehearsals, hanging out with theatre nerds, filling my lungs with air and belting out show tunes. The production's closing number, "I'll Build a Stairway to Paradise," has me in the most thrilling costume of my life. As one of a handful of showgirls, my white ostrich feather, sequin and rhinestone headdress is eighteen inches high and weighs almost two pounds. I have to ascend a railingless flight of stairs sideways and in heels—blinded by stage lights and a bit of actual blindness—while high-kicking and singing, and trying not to look terrified. It's the ultimate test of balance, and if they made physio this fun, I would probably do more physio.

I am the weakest link, the crappiest showgirl on stage. If anyone else had fit the costume, they for sure would have replaced me. If the director knew I had MS, she wouldn't have cast me in this number in the first place.

I try not to sweat it. This isn't Broadway or even Vegas. This is community theatre in Steeltown, and I am so delighted to do it. My showgirl moment is a "fuck you" to MS. It feels like my Everest but better, because I get to do it with a red lip, a beaded bodysuit and a generous round of applause.

One night after a particularly tiring rehearsal, the drummer from the pit band offers to drive me home. I accept gratefully; I'm too tired for the twenty-minute walk. In a moment of vulnerability, I let my guard down and tell him I have MS. I've been hiding it so hard and the lie is exhausting. Drum Guy tells me his sister has MS too, and for a split second I feel relief, like I've confided in someone who gets it.

"You are amazing. Nothing like my sister. She doesn't leave the house; she just talks to her MS friends on the internet all day. She's all doom and gloom." Drum Guy makes his sister sound like a loser and I feel defensive on her behalf. He doesn't get it. My resolve to keep my health status a secret is renewed.

Feeling good with MS, or even just feeling not terrible, comes with a serious side of guilt when MS is the reason I'm not working. The pressure to prove my worth isn't entirely self-imposed. When the new minister at the church where I am the choir's soprano-section lead asks,

"So, what do you do?" I have lots of answers but none of them are what he's after.

When people ask this question, I can never bring myself to say the basic truth, that, well, I paid into a disability insurance plan and then I acquired a disability and made a claim. Of course, the short answer is none of your fucking business, but that feels like an extreme amount of hostility to bring to a man of the cloth. I choke on saying, *I'm on disability*, because I worry the interpretation will be *Oh you're one of those people. Living off the system. A loser.*

I answer the minister's question by talking about singing and the gallery, a recent trip to the farmers' market.

"But what do you do for money?" he clarifies with stunning bluntness. I feel my neck lurch, literally taken aback, even though I could see this coming. Why is what I do for money more interesting than how I spend my time, unless it's to size me up? Of course, once a disclosure of medical retirement has been made, the next question will be either "what's wrong with you?" or "what do you do all day?" Although the former is just nosy, the latter feels like an invitation to defend how I spend my time while the rest of the world is engaged in the morality of work. We talk about earning a living as if being alive doesn't automatically grant us the right to exist.

I call my lawyer cousin, Laura, not because I need a lawyer but because I need to vent.

"I'm feeling good—I'm managing. I'm also feeling judged, like people think that if I have time to volunteer, I should use that time for work." I might think this myself. Though I also believe that volunteering is a more worthwhile contribution to society than whatever I was doing in finance, making money for someone else.

"How many hours are you spending at the gallery?"

"Three-ish. No more than six."

"A day?"

"A week."

"What about the show?"

"The show's over, but it was a few evenings a week for about a month."

"How much sleep did you need today? How much time did you spend dealing with your bladder and bowel? What's your leg pain like?"

"Uhm, badgering the witness?"

"There's a reason why you're not working. Have you considered that's why you feel good?"

"Not everyone thinks like you . . ."

"Fuck 'em. If you have four good hours a day, I don't think it's fair to say that you have to use them working."

I know she's right. I just wish the world agreed.

"Sweetie, what happens when you have the next attack?"

Why is it so hard for me to accept that there will always be a next attack?

17 / The Killing Room

"BRAVA, DIVA!" John beams from behind the piano, as pleased by my Mariah Carey–like whistle tones as if he'd produced them himself.

After my diagnosis I never got back on the bus to see my former singing teacher in Toronto, and when I learned that Canadian baritone and national treasure John Fanning was giving a handful of students private lessons at his studio in nearby Dundas, Ontario, I sat on the intel for months. There was no guarantee he would be interested in taking me on as a student, but more than that, I was afraid to start lessons only to have my heart broken by MS again. I waited until I felt reasonably confident I could commit to weekly lessons and daily practice before I reached out.

When John agreed to take me on as a student, I could barely believe my good fortune, and once I got going, felt like a fool for not signing up sooner. Singing is 360 degrees of physical, spiritual and psychological healing. The hour and half I spend in John's studio on Wednesday nights are the best ninety minutes of my week. Better than therapy. Better than drugs. John Fanning is basically human Prozac. Not only is he ridiculously talented, he is an incredibly generous teacher. He puts no limits on my potential, treating me like a world-class singer without ever letting on that I never could be.

My voice improves by leaps and bounds under John's expert tutelage and eventually I start to get some actual paying gigs. It's not real money, but it is money. Sort of. Money-lite. Enough to sing for my supper, but not enough to cover the mortgage. The difference between singing and being a so-called singer is a lot like the difference between writing and being a writer. My thanks-for-coming-out pay doesn't come close to justifying what I spend on the outfits I perform in, but it's enough to provide the validation that comes with seeing my name on a pay stub with the word *singer* in the subject line. Someone (other than my parents) thinks I have a voice worth listening to.

Ever since MS showed up in my life, I've spent a lot of time feeling frustrated and angry about what my body can't do, but when I'm singing, I feel like *Holy shit, look at what my body* can *do.* I marvel at my high notes, vibrato and breath control. I love the feeling of being able to tell a story with music and to fill a cathedral with sound. The difference between singing and being able to call myself a singer ceases to feel important because I am compensated in far more meaningful ways than tens of dollars. When I'm singing, I feel healed and happy and whole. I am my me-est me. I sing, therefore I am.

And now my ability to sing is being threatened.

LATE ONE NIGHT, a white envelope slides under the front door of our apartment. "That's strange," TB says. "It's addressed to you, but there's no postage." Ten p.m. is a nefarious time to have any kind of correspondence slide under the door unannounced. TB hands me the letter and I tear it open, completely unprepared for what's inside.

"No, no, no, no, no, no, no, this can't be happening."

"What? What does it say?"

"It's from the condo board," I say. "They're threatening legal action against my 'loud opera singing.' Apparently I'm impeding the neighbours' rights to a peaceful existence." I roll my eyes but I feel an existential panic. I can't put a mute on my voice the way I put a mute on my violin when I took up the instrument as a teenager. (And even with the mute, my dad still made me practise in the garage.)

I know my singing is loud. Our open-concept loft has polished concrete floors and twelve-foot ceilings, making it the acoustic equivalent of singing in the shower, exaggerating the fullness of my sound and bothering the fuck out of the philistines.

I practise at least a couple of hours a day but never in the evenings, and certainly not before noon when I'm barely awake. This is communal living; we live smack dab in the middle of the downtown core, where we hear traffic and sirens and sounds of life all day. When I ask my immediate neighbour if anyone has ever complained when he plays his baby grand piano, the answer is no, of course not. How is this different?

I am devastated but determined to find a solution. My well-being, my raison d'être, is at stake. I briefly wonder if I could practise in the underground parking lot before I come up with a better, if somewhat extreme, idea. Fortunately, The Banker's on board.

We hire a contractor, who tells us this is a highly unusual request, but he thinks he can make my dreams come true and convert the closet in the guest room into a soundproof practice room.

The contractor covers the walls of the closet with that squiggly white stuff that sucks up sound. He replaces the flimsy sliding door with drywall and a heavy exterior door. There's no room for my piano, but I could fit a keyboard in there, a music stand, a chair and a mirror. It will be cozy. A room of my own.

The project takes a few days to complete, and when it's finished, The Banker and the contractor go into the hall outside our unit and I enter my new studio to test it out. I sing the loudest, screechiest scales at the top of my register—full voice—and I don't hold back. Ten minutes later the three of us reconvene.

"Nothing."

"Nothing? Not even a hint?"

"Not a whisper. You could scream bloody murder and no one would hear you."

"Thank you, thank you, thank you!" I gush, both to the competent contractor and to my ever-indulgent husband, who supports my increasingly crazy whims and would do just about anything to make me happy. Problem solved.

18 / Employees Only

THE WALK TO MY hair appointment is an ambitious thirty minutes, but it's a beautiful day and I hate the bus. I'm a block away from my destination when I suddenly have to pee. There's no rhyme or reason to when my bladder decides It's Time. Fortunately I'm right outside a Tim Hortons. Well, a mini Tim Hortons. A TiHo. There's a drive-through and a walk-up counter, but no seating. There's nobody at the counter ahead of me, and I silently thank the sweet baby Jesus that the "employees only" bathroom is five feet away. Salvation is within sight.

I start pleading my case. "I will totally buy a carrot muffin, or a water, or whatever, but first can I please use your bathroom? I have MS and it's kind of an emergency."

"Sorry, the bathroom is for employees only." She does not look sorry.

"I know, I just, could you please make an exception? It's medical and I have MS, and, and . . ." I'm blabbering. My hand is pinched between my thighs.

"Let me ask the owner. Sandy? This girl has MS and she wants to use the bathroom." Sandy takes her sweet-ass time wandering over to my side of the counter. I have already peed a bit.

"Oh, you poor thing. I completely understand." Thank God. "My niece has MS."

Great, now please hurry and unlock the door and we can compare notes while I eat that goddamn muffin.

"I can't let you use the staff washroom, though. For insurance purposes."

Now I'm in the bathroom at the Dairy Queen two blocks away, taking deep breaths and trying not to cry as I call the salon to cancel my appointment because I have to go home and wash the brand-new Seven7 jeans I've just baptized. In general, I make an effort not to let myself feel embarrassed or ashamed of my bladder issues. But laying myself bare and being denied help anyway is a deeper kind of humiliation to overcome.

My new disease-modifying drug isn't doing anything to keep my bladder under control. I'm either peeing my pants or I can't pee at all, all day, every day. None of the bladder medications have worked. The patches give me dry mouth and leave glue residue on my sensitive skin. I've got a permanent dark red bruise and chafing on my pelvis from pressing on my lower abdomen in an attempt to manually push the pee out. My bladder is a dictator in charge of all my actions, decisions and plans.

Finally, I'm referred to a urologist. The office is conveniently located down the hall from Dr. Poker Face. Unlike Dr. PF's pink walls and water lily print decor, the urologist's waiting room is full of sports magazines and dudes with prostate cancer. I'm guessing this guy doesn't see a lot of vaginas. At least not professionally. I'm feeling ballsy, pun intended, so I ask how many MS patients he sees. What I really mean is, how many female MS patients he sees, and I take a lighthearted dig at his *Motorcycle Digest*–heavy reading room.

The urologist assures me he can handle MS. He listens carefully to my complaints, quotes Shakespeare and then recommends we do something called a urodynamics test. I don't ask too many questions about what's involved in a urodynamics test, because now we're talking about literature and opera, and maybe this guy's not a bro after all.

I'm feeling vulnerable and exposed in a paper gown, my feet in stirrups. The operating room is nothing if not well lit, and the miner's light strapped to Dr. Bard's forehead feels like overkill. He prepares to take a look deep inside my bladder with a camera that, once introduced, feels like a repurposed Elizabethan quill. Various substances are then pumped into my bladder: water, soap—gas, for some reason. It's painful, and I hate that I'm alive for any of it. I wouldn't say I was tricked, but perhaps I was given a false sense of security from Dr. Bard's cognoscente vibes. If anyone even whispers "urodynamics" to you, call your fastest-driving friend to come and get you immediately. Urodynamics is not some Eurotrash dance club. Though you will wish you had thought to take Molly.

The test proves what we already know: MS is fucking up my bladder. Dr. Bard explains that the bladder is like a balloon. MS causes retention;

when my brain tells my body it's time to pee, my body sends the call straight to voice mail. The reason I'm having incontinence is that eventually the bladder gets so overfull that the overflow has no place to go but onto my crisp white bedsheets. Since I'm releasing only the overflow, my bladder never fully empties, and that is why I have to pee every eighteen minutes. Mystery solved, but what's the solution? Dr. Bard suggests intermittent self-catheterization. ISC.

THE BANKER LEAVES the apartment and I make him take the dog, because I don't want any witnesses, human or otherwise. A nurse is coming twice a day for the next five days to teach me how to self-catheterize. The word *catheter* is too scary to say, and I can tell by the look on anyone's face when I mention it that it's also too scary to hear. Maybe if I refer to the tool as Cathy, the word won't get stuck in my throat.

The training session should take only an hour, but I don't want The Banker anywhere near this version of me, and three hours feels like a good buffer in case the nurse is chatty. I already had to explain to my husband *who has a biology degree* that Urethra lives in her own zip code, one that is separate and unique from her neighbour, Vagina, and that's enough medicalization of my lady parts to last a lifetime. Even so, he'd better come back with a present. This is a Medical Milestone Day. I'm not interested in sewing a patch that says I've earned my "self-catheterizer" badge onto my sick-person sash, but it still feels like I deserve some recognition for what feels like a pretty big deal. Diamonds, maybe, but I'll settle for flowers.

The nurse asks where the bedroom is and I know that lately I've been doing some of my best peeing in bed, but the whole point of making friends with Cathy is to stop peeing in inappropriate places.

The nurse is not chatty, and has little patience for my nervousness. She pulls back the duvet, lays down a pad and tells me to take off my pants. She doesn't close the curtains despite my floor-to-ceiling windows.

It shouldn't take an industry just to be able to pee, and yet here we are. The nurse has an enormous box of supplies that reinforce how unnatural all of this is. She produces a bedpan, a mirror, several packages of long plastic tubes, gloves, gauze (for some reason)—are those scissors?—and packages of lubricant.

I prop my head up with pillows and put on the disposable gloves. The nurse then shows me how to put lubricant on the clear tube that feels threateningly long. She holds a mirror between my legs, and tells me to find my urethra and guide Cathy into my bladder. "Like tapping a keg," I joke, but she doesn't laugh. Probably never been invited to any keg parties.

The mirror is useless. I'm not blind, but I'm *legally* blind, which basically means I can see enough to function but I can't safely drive a car or locate a pin-sized hole in a haystack via reflection. When it feels like things couldn't get any more uncomfortable, the nurse asks if I have a flashlight. Suddenly I'm fourteen again, frustrated on the floor with the Tampax instructions unfolded in front of me, wondering how women ever manage to get the hang of their own impossible anatomy. At least when I was fourteen I didn't have to figure it out in front of an audience.

The coaching is ridiculous. The nurse can't see through my hand to tell me where to go. When at last the tube disappears into my body, my triumph is short-lived. Nothing happens. Wrong orifice. Cathy has been contaminated and we have to start again, lubing up a new sterile Cathy-clone. When I finally find my urethra, I feel a burst of pride. Like I've accomplished something athletic. A hole in one. Eventually. Moments later my bladder is empty and a choir of angels sings. I'd forgotten how satisfying a truly empty bladder feels. It's not quite bliss, but it's close.

On day three, my potty training moves from the bedroom to the bathroom. It's actually easier to find my urethra sitting up, and I feel annoyed that my training didn't start out this way. It occurs to me that my nurse has probably never personally made friends with Cathy, and that she might have been a better teacher if she had.

It's a couple of weeks before I completely get the hang of it. And just as I mastered tampons as a teen, it's not long before I can self-catheterize drunk and in the dark. Any time I have to pee, I just tap the keg and get on with it. I don't even have to think about it. Because my bladder never gets stressed and overfull, I stop having accidents entirely. Like, 100 percent. Over. It never happens.

Cathy has liberated me. If it were up to me, we'd stop using the eagle to symbolize freedom and replace it with a catheter and a sweaty unhooked bra, but months later I'm once again filled with cynicism and antibiotic-resistant bacteria. I realize that Cathy's more frenemy than bestie. Introducing plastic and synthetic lube into an orifice that's not meant to be entered means I'm still getting UTIs. I mostly become aware of these infections on Fridays at 4 p.m., after my family doctor's office has stopped taking calls for the weekend. In the interest of efficiency, I start to wonder if I can order a petri dish and learn how to do my own cultures. I'm sure there's a way to order antibiotics from Mexico.

Eventually I discover that the hospital-grade catheters I've been using are not my only option; they're just the most affordable. (I will never stop being frustrated by just how much I have to figure out on my own with this disease.) The cheap plastic and low polish of the low-rent catheters can chafe the urethra and invite bacteria.

I upgrade to a mini-mascara-sized, pre-lubricated tool I can take on the road. Cathy 2.0 is fancy. Fortunately I have insurance because I'm paying exponentially more than I've ever paid to even the bougiest *dame pipi* in a Paris public washroom, and Cathy doesn't come with a complimentary hand towel or a spritz of off-brand hair spray. *Oh, is that a Chanel bag? How charming. I flush $4.61 down the toilet every time I pee.*

Learning to cath feels like one of the best things I've ever done for my MS, but I'm still pissy, at least metaphorically. The thing that proved to be a solution was made out to be a problem. I'm pissed that I wasn't offered Cathy three years ago. That I had to suffer through so many useless medications that only caused side effects. Positioning self-catheterization as a last resort gave me end-of-the-road energy, when it could have been sold as "let's try this tool" instead.

I arrive at my follow-up appointment with Dr. Bard ready to rant about my frustrations, but I lose steam when I discover that his waiting room is now stocked with issues of *Vogue* and *Vanity Fair.*

19 / Outed

IT'S A STAGE DOOR DAY, which is my absolute favourite kind of day; plus, it's Christmastime, so there's basically no reining in my enthusiasm. I've reached Peak Joy. My outfit, a bubble-hem high-low strapless gown designed to show off my shoes and shoulders, matches my jubilant mood. My brand-new black patent Louboutins are about to make their debut with the Aradia Ensemble at the Glenn Gould Theatre in Toronto. I'll be singing Handel's *Messiah*. My shoes will be singing my praises.

Stage Door Days start with self-indulgent Stage Door mornings. Hair, nails, lemon water, maybe a massage. *Namaste.* I try to keep myself grounded as I prepare for centre-of-attention time. I don't suffer from pre-performance jitters, but I do have to keep the butterflies at bay lest I have a repeat of the time I was so excited to be headlining Mozart's *Requiem* that I had to make a stop at emerg to have some chest pain checked out before the concert. An ECG confirmed I was medically fit to sing, and the doctor sent me away with a prescription to slow my roll, eat a banana, calm the fuck down.

Phase Two of Stage Door Days starts once I've crossed the threshold of the stage door in question. I have a quick convo with the butterflies to let them know that there's nothing life-threatening about the compounded energy of the other singers, the last-minute lipstick and lip trills, the cheesy prayer circles while the orchestra tunes to A440. *Listen, you butterfly bitches, I'm glad you're here, but stay in my tummy where you belong. No need to get the heart involved.* Then, the blur of performance, followed by applause, flowers, kudos, a boozy afterparty and the decision of whether to linger in post-performance insomnia, smiling stupidly at the ceiling, or to insist on sleep by drowning my hyper-arousal in champagne. Either way, I'm not taking off my makeup until tomorrow.

Ranking almost as high as the high I get from performing is a day spent in Paris, where even a bad day is better than a good day anywhere else. I don't even need a full day to get a decent Paris buzz—a two-hour layover at Charles de Gaulle can be an effective microdose if I plan my airport shopping right: a jar of Edmond Fallot Dijon, an éclair from La Maison du Chocolat, a foulard from Galeries Lafayette if there's time.

I know there's nothing interesting or original about my love for Paris, but being in Paris fills my body with its own excited butterflies. Hearty ones too, because I feed them pastries, wine and cheese. They don't get any vegetables (unless you count *frites*, which I absolutely do). If these *papillons* ever make it to my heart, I will need that ECG after all.

A trip to Paris is always special but my most recent visit to the city of lights two months ago was especially memorable for the day I climbed the thirteen hundred steps to the bell tower at Notre-Dame Cathedral to high-five Quasimodo himself. It was a particularly poignant achievement after being too weak to do it just a few years ago. From the Galerie des Chimères, I reached out to touch the eight-hundred-year-old monsters and gazed at the Seine, Sacré-Coeur, Saint-Sulpice, la tour Eiffel. My accomplishment felt epic, like I'd come back not quite from the dead, but the dead-adjacent. Just like singing, I reclaimed a precious experience that I thought MS had permanently taken. As I scanned the city looking for the Arc de triomphe, I thought to myself, *Damn right, motherfuckers, I have triumphed.*

A slaying of this magnitude deserved a proper trophy. The gargoyles were not for sale. Since I wanted to thank my feet for carrying me up and all over Paris, shoes seemed a fitting solution. Not sensible shoes, of course. Victory shoes. Shoes that scream celebration. And that's how I ended up at Christian Louboutin's famous flagship store maxing out my credit card on the scarlet-soled stilettos I'll be wearing on stage tonight.

I haven't deluded myself into thinking I'll be able to wear a heel this high forever. I simply decided to take full and extravagant advantage of the fact that I can wear these statement shoes now. The statement of course being: *va te faire foutre, MS*.

Although the shoes demand attention, *Fuck MS* is more of a whisper; something I keep to myself. There's no reason the other singers, and especially the conductor, need to know about my condition. This is a professional gig. I'm still new on the scene, and my unreliable health doesn't feel like the kind of intel that will make me seem like an asset.

Backstage, everyone clocks my shoe game. The girls want to try them on (absolutely not), the basses roll their eyes, the tenors get it. When I walk onstage, I swear I hear someone in the audience gasp. It's the appropriate reaction. Artsy, fancy, gay, these are my people. Pitched forward, tits out, I feel like a goddess. I feel so good that the only reasonable thing left to do is sing.

After the concert I slip into something less formal but no less considered—knee-high boots and a 1960s-style printed minidress with a red chevron print and two white pompoms around the neck, because it's Christmas. I deposit my gown at coat check, but I'm not letting my shoes leave my sight. My Louboutins, tucked safely into their red dust bag, are stashed in the tote bag beside me.

"Let's get another bottle, shall we?" It's not a question. Kevin, Aradia's Irish American artistic director, knows how to party. I'm on a post-performance high myself, and a bit of a red wine one too.

"What happened to your heels?" Snarky Bass asks when he sees me.

"Oh, those are just part-time shoes," I say laughing. "Heels like that aren't sustainable."

"Sopranos," he says, and rolls his eyes again.

"I think they're fabulous," Kevin says. "It's ballet shoes you have to be careful about." Someone launches into a story about the blackened toes of a dancer they once dated. Before the table finishes the next bottle of wine, the conversation has taken a deep dive into footwear-related trauma: ingrown toenails, broken metatarsals, stepping on tent pegs. Even the city's coolest culture-makers like a good gross-out story.

Eager to contribute, I decide to share the harrowing tale of how my French former boyfriend ice-skated over my finger when I was seventeen. The story has everything: international intrigue, a jealous rival who intentionally crashed into us as we skated together holding hands, a potential career as a violinist cut short by a severed (then reattached) digit, a romance torn apart by guilt and shame; it's practically Shakespearean.

I open my mouth to speak but in a rare example of The Banker getting a word in before me, TB starts to speak too. He's probably going to talk about the time he stepped on a tack. Boring and predictable. There's no drama in this anecdote, no plot. He didn't need stitches and a tetanus shot. He didn't hallucinate a terrifying nurse with a syringe the size of a baby's arm after a hefty dose of narcotics. Still, I yield the floor because that's what marriage is about.

"That reminds me of the time I had one of Ardra's needles stuck in my toe," he starts. Shit. This is not the story I was expecting. "We were in Montreal, and she was about to shoo . . . shoot—" He stops cold, then looks at me, panicked.

I raise my eyebrows, with a look that says, *I can't help you; you're on your own.* My artificial smile communicates the subtext: *This a colossal fuck-up. You owe me big time.* TB is about to tell the story about the time my MS was being treated with subcutaneous interferon and my auto-injector failed. After slamming the device into my thigh, like I'd done hundreds of times before, nothing happened. Ever the hero, The Banker had tried to intervene. Wearing nothing but boxers, he'd stood barefoot in the bathroom of our hotel room trying to dislodge the loaded syringe from the stuck device. When he was finally able to open the auto-injector, the needle flew up into the air with the grace of an Olympic diver, before gravity took over and stuck the landing directly in the middle of TB's barefooted big toe. Mesmerized, and not yet in pain or sensing danger, like a psycho, he yelled, "Quick! Get the camera." As far as medical misadventures go, I don't deny that Needlegate is a solid story, but without the MS context, "drug-filled syringe in the toe" sounds a lot like the mishap of a junkie.

"Not needle, but, uhm, like a . . ." The Banker's blubbering attempt to bail on the truth only makes things worse. His sketchy plot holes reinforce the *Are these two on heroin?* narrative. I'm tempted to out his third nipple, but I respect boundaries, and that's his story to tell. In any case, it's too late. The table is hooked and wants to hear how *Pulp Fiction* turns out.

"Actually, I have MS," I say, in the chillest, it's-no-big-deal way I can muster, knowing the truth won't set me free. If all the world's a stage, I've been playing young and healthy, someone capable you can count on, who's not under the constant threat of episodic illness. My secret's out, but the role I've been cast in has only shifted. The truth is only palatable if I'm a certain kind of patient (positive, self-sufficient, kick-ass, but not so kick-ass that people think I'm faking). I slip my hand in my bag and touch my Louboutins, like a talisman. "Actually, my husband's charming anecdote is about my MS medication. It's an injection that keeps my disease stable. Perfectly legal. Not even fun." Ha ha.

"Really?" says Kevin, with the usual surprise of someone who thinks I look "normal." "You have MS?" I do a half-nod, half-shrug to reinforce my "no biggie" narrative. Kevin decides whether or not I'll get hired for this ensemble again. It's not the time to enlighten the masses about the realities of invisible illness.

"But," Kevin continues—wide-eyed and confounded—"but, you have so much energy!"

It's not true, but I'm glad he thinks so.

20 / I Forget You Have MS

I'VE BEEN KEEPING MY DIAGNOSIS on the down-low for a number of years now, but of course there are people in my inner circle who know all about my condition. From time to time, one of my friends or even someone in my family will say some version of "sometimes I forget you have MS." The observation is meant to be a compliment and, for a long time, that's exactly how I received it.

There's something intoxicating about "passing" as someone who isn't defined by chronic illness. Staying silent means I can be Ardra, instead of Ardra-with-MS.

It's not just me. More than one-third of people living with MS keep their diagnosis classified. But keeping secrets is stressful, and in addition to being accidentally outed from time to time, MS tries to reveal itself in ways that those of us who live with it don't always recognize as our "tells." More than once, I've been asked about my fancy walk, or why the fonts on my phone are so big you can see them from space.

It doesn't help that I'm not good at intrigue. I talk *a lot* and am not exactly known for being the mysterious type. Passing for non-disabled takes effort, and can lead to strange behaviours that I haven't yet figured out how to mitigate. Like, the time I was out for lunch with a new friend from the art gallery. At the time, I was still learning to self-catheterize and spent forty-five minutes in the bathroom looking for my urethra. When I finally came back to the table, I offered absolutely no explanation for my extended absence. My friend probably thought I had diarrhea, but then I ordered dessert.

There was also the time I'd been hired to sing for a production of *Riverdance,* with a live band. I lost my balance at a rehearsal and landed flat on the drum kit. Very rock and roll. I apologized profusely, but gave no reason for my sudden collapse. The band probably thought I was drunk, and that still seemed better to me than sharing the truth about my MS.

Then there was the European choir tour, and, like everyone else, this time I actually was drunk a lot of the time. Tour bus–induced motion sickness, combined with the amount of rest and the number of early nights I needed, led to rumours that I was pregnant—rumours I didn't bother to correct. I was more comfortable being thought of as reckless and irresponsible than I was in copping to MS.

The concept of "passing" has various social contexts, most notably within racialized and LGBTQIA+ communities. People with MS are marginalized in different ways, but have often felt the need to hide an identity over which they have no control. Many fear how disclosure of an MS diagnosis will impact careers, relationships and safety. People with MS risk being isolated, stigmatized and seen as less-than. Just like racism and homophobia, ableism exists.

For many with MS, the "should I or shouldn't I" decision can cause anxiety and depression. I know of at least one woman with relapsing MS—a doctor—who told her spouse she was diagnosed with a less serious condition out of fear that her partner would leave her. Of all the burdens of this disease, shouldering it alone, without the support of loved ones, adds a whole new layer of hardship.

It's not enough to be told that the world will understand and that the law is on our side. Because, is the law *really* on our side when there are systems in place that keep disabled bodies out of sight? When inaccessibility is standard, medications and medical equipment aren't affordable and people with disabilities regularly have to fight for benefits and opportunities?

It can be terrifying to tell someone in a position of power or influence that you have MS. "Able bodies are better than disabled bodies" is something you can still say out loud and not get cancelled. You might even believe it yourself.

It's equally acceptable to make disability the butt of the joke. If you think I'm being dramatic, let me remind you of TikTok's viral New Teacher Challenge where parents—PARENTS—pretend to introduce kids to their teachers over Zoom using photos of adults with congenital facial differences and other disabilities. The kids often respond with fear and/or tears while their parents and TikTok viewers laugh mightily.

The desire to be included is powerful. Human beings have a need to fit in. Disability is the largest minority in the world, and yet we haven't found safety in numbers, let alone pride in identity. So many people are afraid of being "found out" and seen as damaged, broken, sick, less-than. Maybe this sounds hyperbolic, but it's hard to acknowledge membership in a group that almost no one wants to be a part of. It's difficult to claim status in a society that has a hierarchy of bodies, and that values productivity and so-called perfection above all else.

And so, if we are able, some of us hide our MS from strangers, coworkers, even from the people we depend on for survival. Sure, passing has its privileges, but I'm starting to see the damage passing can do. For one thing, keeping quiet leaves us to fend for ourselves, without accommodations. Lack of support can lead to frustration, fatigue and a reduced ability to perform the tasks of daily living. But keeping quiet can have deeper consequences too.

When we don't feel safe enough to disclose our MS, we end up reinforcing the message that we have something shameful to hide. Even the language around sharing a diagnosis as something to be *disclosed* suggests there's something sneaky going on, something that needs confessing.

Coming out with MS is a process. It doesn't just happen once, but over and over again, depending on the situation. I don't owe anyone an explanation of how I move through the world, especially when there's enough evidence to prove disclosure is not always in my best interest. But, as long as MS is my sick little secret, I will never truly be free to be myself. My sense of security and safety depends on maintaining a lie. When the status quo goes unquestioned, saying "that's not me; I'm not one of those people" perpetuates the stigma around chronic illness. It suggests that disability is a choice, a lifestyle one can simply decide to opt out of.

"Sometimes I forget you have MS" suggests that I am the "right" kind of patient. Someone who doesn't complain too much or ask for too much help. "Sometimes I forget you have MS" is only truly a compliment if remembering that I have MS is an insult. Saying "I have MS but don't worry; it doesn't really affect me" is not the same as having the confidence to say "I have MS and I have a right to be meaningfully included."

Although an MS diagnosis is still perceived as a liability, I'm starting to appreciate that one of the unexpected burdens of this illness is to recognize social injustice and to try to resist it—try to change things. Not just for myself but for the communities I am a part of. Being accepted for who I am starts with accepting myself.

21 / Lie-beration Therapy

THE MS WORLD is wigging out about what's been dubbed chronic cerebrospinal venous insufficiency (CCSVI). When *w5*, a TV news program, breaks the story, it's must-see TV for everyone who loves anyone who has MS. The show dedicates a full twenty-two-minute deep dive into Italian vascular surgeon Paolo Zamboni's research. Zamboni doesn't use the word *cure*, but claims to have completely reversed his wife's MS symptoms with a novel but simple procedure. His theory is that reduced blood flow from the brain, due to blocked veins in the head and neck, causes iron deposits to accumulate and fuck shit up. Zamboni reasons that opening up the veins with an angioplasty-type procedure is the answer to MS.

w5 isn't winning any Peabody Awards, but it's 2009, and I don't think too hard about what qualifies Lloyd Robertson to validate the story. Robertson is a serious journalist, an officer of the Order of Canada and the nation's Favourite News Anchor, 1998 *and* 1999. Robertson doesn't use the phrase *fuck shit up* to explain the biology of MS, and when he says "scientific breakthrough," it's easy to believe him.

w5's production is slick. It's full of doctors tossing out words like *irrefutable*, *paradigm shift* and *dramatic results*. There are tearful testimonials from patients who claim they've been given back their lives and that they've forgotten what it feels like to have MS. There's enough B-roll footage of before-and-after miracles backed up by MRI and Doppler scans of blocked veins that by the end of the broadcast, I can't move or speak or look anyone in the eye because I'm convinced that if I so much as exhale, I will wake up from what has to be a dream.

On the other hand, even if Zamboni's not-a-cure is curing Italians in his research trial, I can't help but feel like it won't matter—not for me. It will take years of studies before the procedure is available. Years during which I will continue to rack up damage and disability. The only thing worse than no cure at all is the cure that exists but is just out of reach.

FOURTEEN MONTHS AFTER Lloyd Robertson's compelling TV segment, it's the ten-year anniversary of my MS diagnosis, and it's a loaded milestone. Ten was the magic number of years I was told I would probably have before my MS would transition from "relapsing remitting" to "secondary progressive": the scary stage when attacks slow down but recovery is no longer possible.

Ten years ago, when I was issued this life sentence, I imagined what it would be like to be in a wheelchair at thirty-three. I told myself that thirty-three was pretty old anyway.

What a fucking twat.

Today, I am telling my MS not to get too comfortable. The media has coined Dr. Zamboni's treatment "liberation therapy" and even though the phrase makes me throw up in my mouth, I am nonetheless getting on a plane tomorrow to have the procedure in Poland, where a clinic in Katowice is treating international MS patients.

Darcy is fully convinced that CCSVI is the answer. She's on her way to a clinic in Mexico to have the procedure herself. Despite the conviction of my friends and family that Zamboni's procedure will fix us, I try not to have too many expectations. I don't know if this surgery will stop my MS from progressing, but I know I have to try. For the first time in ten years, when it comes to my health, I have something that feels like hope.

I'm making this trip without my doctor's blessing or knowledge. Like most conventional neurologists, Dr. Poker Face isn't convinced CCSVI is a thing. I don't want to be judged or condescended to, but more than that, I don't want to risk being dismissed as a patient, so I keep my mouth shut.

Meanwhile, my friends and family marvel at how brave I am to take a chance on an experimental procedure in a foreign country. *Experimental procedure* sounds like some Dr. Frankenstein–level risk taking, but it's really just an angioplasty. I mean, how different can veins and arteries be? Plus, I'm a seasoned traveller. To me, the opportunity to eat authentic pierogies and sample Polish vodka is a perk. My decision is the opposite of brave. I am completely motivated by fear. Brave would be accepting a future where I am more disabled.

Our journey to Poland does not go smoothly. Our indirect flight is thwarted by an airline strike and The Banker and I are forced to be flexible and change plans a number of times. Eventually we end up at a train station in Katowice. It's a post-industrial town, where in January, everything looks like it's in black and white.

We are met by a guy named Piotr, who ushers us into a Euromedics van, where five other medical tourists are waiting. Barb from Manitoba is here with her husband. She's just off a twenty-hour flight but is somehow bubbling with energy. Helen is from Nova Scotia and makes it clear that, unlike Barb, she's not interested in making friends. Helen and Barb will both be having the procedure the same day as me.

The remaining passengers are a couple from Holland. The husband's name sounds like *fuck* with two *u*'s and an *e* on the end. Fuucke. Fuucke was treated here four months ago and is a true believer. He tells us he spent the summer walking normally, but that he's here for a tune-up because apparently veins can re-stenose. He insists my vision will be 20/20, maybe even better than 20/20 by the end of the week. I don't believe him but I let it slide. I don't dare ask the universe for improvements. I vow to be satisfied if "liberation therapy" just keeps me from getting worse.

Piotr drives us to the business hotel that's part of the international CCSVI medical tourism package we purchased, and it's obvious that he's proud to be part of a program that one-ups Canada's legendary health-care system. He explains that, throughout the week, we will see a neurologist, and have physiotherapy, massages, an MRI, an eye exam and an ECG. Most of this will take place on-site at the hotel. It's like an all-inclusive beach vacay, but with less sun and unlimited cabbage.

My first pre-surgery appointment is an ECG on the eleventh floor. A pimply kid in jeans and a T-shirt opens the repurposed hotel suite's door and ushers me in without telling me his name. I ask the boy when the technician will be here. He doesn't seem to understand the question and leads me to the exam table.

"Take off shirt and bra," he says.

So, I guess he's the technician? I look around for a hospital gown, but there's nothing in sight. "Can I get a sheet or a towel or something?" He looks at me like I've asked for drugs or weapons. The room feels uncomfortably well lit. I guess we're doing this.

"You look like you're fifteen," I say, as the boy places electrodes on my naked torso.

"Thank you," he replies, as if this were a compliment and not an accusation.

When the electrodes are in place, he hands me a small towel that I assume is to cover myself with, but the towel won't cover both of my breasts. Maybe if I smoosh my boobs together, I could get decent nipple coverage, but that feels like the wrong move. I place the towel over the boob that's closest to the boy technician, without asking for anything else, because somehow now I feel like I'm the one being weird, and anyway, I don't want to prolong the experience. I've had my share of vulnerable medical moments, but this feels like I'm being punked or am inadvertently starring in some low-budget, soundtrack-less Polish porno.

Thankfully, the ECG is over quickly. I use the towelette to wipe away the electrode goo, knowing I'm missing most of it but anxious to get dressed and get out. I'm almost at the door when Polish Doogie Howser tells me that I must repeat the ECG when I go back to Canada.

"Was there something abnormal?" I ask.

"Nothing worry. Voff Parkinson."

What the fuck? "Parkinson's?" I question, certain I must have heard wrong.

"Ya. Nothing worry."

"PARKINSON'S DISEASE?" Now my eyes are bugging out as I try to understand.

"That is the name of condition."

I feel myself go pale. Doogie Howser starts writing and then hands me a low-quality photocopied leaflet with his photo and credentials. His real name is Jarosław and he's a recent graduate of "Medical High School." Medical High School must have a comprehensive curriculum, because according to the leaflet, Jarosław is also the massage therapist.

On the back of the paper he has written in all caps: MORE DISTANT DIAGNOSTIC WITH VIEW TO CONFIRMING THE TEAM OF THE SICK WOLF-PARKINSON'S WHIT'S.

I snatch the paper out of his hand and race to the elevator. My heart is pounding. Impossibly, the elevator is playing the chorus of "Everything's Gonna Be Alright." Fuck you, elevator. I cannot have MS and Parkinson's. I cannot. It will not be alright.

Bursting into our hotel room, I throw the note and my water bottle on the floor and head straight to the bathroom because the only issue that's more pressing than my pending mortality is my need to pee.

Moments later I emerge, pick up the paper and grab The Banker. This is 2011, early smart phone days, and I don't have a device in my pocket to enable a quick consult with Dr. Google. "Come with me," I tell TB in a tone of voice he doesn't question. I don't say anything on our way to the communal computer in the lobby. Because what would I say? *I just need to quickly ask the internet if my life is over*? The rational part of me must realize that Parkinson's disease cannot possibly be diagnosed by a ten-minute hotel room ECG performed by a teenaged graduate of Medical High School, but the rational part of me does not, in this moment, exist. I've been through the trauma of a devastating diagnosis before. I know that life can change in a heartbeat.

I go to the Mayo Clinic website and type Jarosław's words—WOLF-PARKINSON'S WHIT'S—into the search engine while TB stands behind me, watching the screen in confusion. The results bring up a condition called Wolff-Parkinson-White syndrome, WPW. It's not the same as Parkinson's disease. Not at all. WPW is a congenital heart defect and I've never been happier to have a broken heart.

I quickly determine that WPW sounds manageable, even benign, although sudden death is technically possible. Relief washes over me. Sudden death is statistically unlikely, and anyway sounds better than the slow decline I imagine happens with actual Parkinson's (at least in my current state of mind), and who the hell was this Parkinson anyway? How many diseases is this guy named after? Still, I am shaken. I feel far from home. Not yet up to speed and unaware of the bullet I've managed to dodge, TB just looks bewildered.

At 6 a.m. the day of the procedure, we pile into Piotr's van. Helen is quietly working on her resting bitch face, while Barb seems to think we're on our way to Disneyland. Piotr takes us to a run-down hospital; the exterior looks institutional, like a repurposed prison.

Once inside, I am abruptly separated from The Banker and ushered into a room with Barb and Helen, where we are hastily undressed by three nurses who do not speak a word of English. The nurse charged with starting my IV yells directives at me in Polish. I consult the cheat sheet of translations we were given. It has phrases like "the blood which you can see in plastic tube is normal sign" and "I need to have a bowel." Of course I don't expect everyone to be able to speak English, and I understand that I am a guest in this country, but it's a particular kind of vulnerability to put yourself in the care of people you can't reliably communicate with. Even if I did need to have a bowel, I have no idea how to pronounce "*Muszę się załatwić*."

Our room has three single beds and an ensuite bathroom. There are no curtains separating our beds, but the room has a door that closes and a window that opens. We can see a courtyard with an old World War II helicopter and a big black dog roaming around.

Once we are gowned up, The Banker is allowed to come to our room. Dr. Simka arrives shortly after with a portable Doppler ultrasound—a machine that measures blood flow—and now I appreciate the lack of privacy, because I want to hear everyone's results. Helen and Barb both have at least one blocked vein. When Dr. Simka performs my ultrasound, I watch the results pop up on the screen. The blood is flowing through my left jugular. It's not gushing, but it looks normal, healthy. I'm relieved when the doctor moves the wand to my right jugular. The difference in blood flow is dramatic. The fat vein is clearly blocked, and I can see the blood barfing back up into my brain. That the doctor can see a problem means there's something to fix.

Helen is the first to be treated. She's gone for about forty-five minutes, and when they bring her back, she's loopy and half-conscious. Her legs are bound together, and on the count of what I assume is Polish "one, two, three," she is flung from the gurney onto her bed. It looks and sounds violent. Barb and I exchange nervous looks but Helen just laughs. It's reassuring to know Helen is capable of laughter.

Minutes later, Barb is being wheeled out for her procedure. When they bring her back, she lands with the same disturbing crash as she is flung onto her bed. Like Helen, she doesn't seem to notice.

I decide to pee one more time before it's my turn. But nobody comes. Two hours later, The Banker is pacing, and nervous about why I haven't been treated yet. He goes looking for answers from someone who speaks English and finds out that my procedure is delayed because a patient has come in with an emergency, and it's all hands on deck at the tiny hospital.

I've been hooked up to an over-enthusiastic saline IV for six hours now, and I've never peed so often in my life. I'm hungry and tired and the longer I'm forced to wait, the more I start to convince myself that this is a mistake and I should bail. But Helen and Barb's drugs have worn off and they are eagerly comparing notes. Helen's procedure seems to have given her a whole new personality, and it occurs to me that her stand-offishness may have actually been nerves. She's relaxed and chatty now, and it's comforting to see both of my roommates doing well.

At 5 p.m. I'm finally taken to the operating room. Once inside, I start to shake. My teeth are chattering. My gown is removed and I am left stark naked and freezing cold on the operating table while my groin gets painted with iodine. For a notoriously Catholic country, they sure don't prioritize modesty in medical situations.

I make a point of being as charming as possible. I'm worried that the surgeon is wrecked from the emergency patient that railroaded the day and that mistakes will be made. I tell him I like his Buddy Holly glasses and then empathize that he must be tired. I ask how the emergency patient is doing. Buddy Holly sees through me and kindly tells me not to worry: he is fresh and I am his first patient. The glasses, he adds, are less fashion and more surgical protective eyewear. Oh.

Despite my relief, I'm still shaking all over and stressing over how anyone could safely perform surgery on a body in motion. When I start to feel giddy and groggy with whatever has been added to my IV, I'm determined to stay as alert as possible. I want to remember every detail. Buddy Holly's English is excellent and I ask him to talk to me throughout the procedure.

My right groin area is frozen before a camera is sent up all the way to my right jugular. Buddy Holly confirms the blockage and proceeds to open it with a balloon. It hurts, and he offers to stop. I can barely speak or swallow because there's a camera in my jugular, but I manage to say no; as long as it's safe and normal for this to hurt, then do what you have to do. The balloon stays open for four minutes, so I guess it's true that one can endure anything for four minutes. (Later, The Banker confirms this by saying that he endured four minutes of *Jackass* in German on the hotel room's TV last night.)

The balloon deflates and the pain begins to subside but then there's a sudden painful pop in my ear. I yelp.

"Ear?" I don't know how he knew (because he's the doctor, duh). My eustachian tubes are going crazy, crackling. Buddy Holly says the left jugular is smooth sailing, that it's as clear as the highway from Toronto to Montreal. Clearly he's never driven on the 401, but I know what he means. Finally, he goes for the azygos vein and I feel a mild discomfort in the middle of my chest. There is no blockage. I am done. Buddy Holly congratulates me for being so tough.

The nurses quickly rock me back and forth as they wrap me in a thick bandage like a mummy, then cover me with a blanket. Moments later I can tell they've added something good to my IV, because finally I stop shaking. I'm wheeled to my shared room and flung onto my bed just as oblivious to the toss as Helen and Barb had been.

Now I have to lie flat for six hours so that I don't bleed to death. Barb and Helen are sound asleep. The Banker has gone back to the hotel so that I can rest. When they finally cut the dressing off, it's close to midnight. I get up to pee and change into pyjamas only to discover that my thighs are still coated in iodine. I guess that's why we were told to bring a towel, which I did not. I am so tired, but I spend the next half-hour with soap and subpar paper towels trying to wash it away.

When I finally crawl into bed the room is quiet and dark. The window is open and the fresh air feels good on my face. Every now and then I hear the big black dog bark and it's more comforting than annoying. It occurs to me that this open-window environment is actually far more civilized and conducive to healing than that of any Canadian hospital room I've ever spent the night in.

It's over. I did it. All I can do now is wait and see. It's January 20, 2011. Tomorrow is my birthday.

IN THE WEEKS to come I'm peppered with questions about the procedure, and I've never felt more pressure to give the "right" answer, the one that satisfies, the one that says, "it worked!"

But eighteen months later, there are new lesions showing on my MRI. Like Fuucke, I return to Poland to see if I've re-stenosed, praying that I've re-stenosed because that will mean there's something we can do.

This time, we are met at the airport by Aleksy and his girlfriend, Anna. They both look like they stayed up all night partying, got up, had sex without showering, then came to get us without brushing their teeth or hair. The Euromedics van has been upgraded to a Mercedes, but when we get inside, there are no other patients, just garbage, blankets and takeout containers.

I'm taken to a brand-new medical facility that feels more like a luxury hotel. My private room has a wall-mounted flat-screen TV, a pillow-top mattress and a down-filled duvet. The bougie new hospital was largely financed by the massive influx of Canadian MS patients, but it's eerily empty. When I was here last, Euromedics was treating an average of seventeen people a week. Now they say two patients a week is considered good.

In 2013, four years after Zamboni busted onto the scene, the debunking of his theory is a top news story. By 2017, Zamboni himself will conclude that venous angioplasty is ineffective and not recommended for treatment of MS. Smug neurologists can't resist saying "I told you so" at every opportunity without ever seeming to consider how they, along with pharmaceutical companies, may have contributed to the erosion of trust that drove roughly five thousand Canadians to step outside of the multi-billion-dollar MS industry that has failed to come up with anything better than high-risk, high-side-effect, high-cost, under-effective medications that do nothing to address the underlying cause of MS, and travel to places like Mexico, Belarus and Russia in the hopes that something else just might save our legs—or our lives.

22 / How Low Can You Go?

"IMRE IS HERE TO SEE YOU. SHALL I SEND HIM UP?" the front desk concierge asks over the phone.

Fuck. He's early. I head to the bathroom to splash cold water on my face so that my vocal coach/accompanist won't be able to tell I'm barely awake, then remind myself not to say "fuck" for the next ninety minutes. Imre's Hungarian-Catholic ears bleed whenever he hears the F-word, so I try to use it less when he's around.

"C'mon in," I yell from the bathroom when I hear a gentle knock at the door. "I'll be right out." Imre's sitting at the piano when I emerge, a stack of scores piled on the bench next to him. He's tinkling the keys and tapping the sticky damper pedal, a passive-aggressive reminder for me to have The Banker WD-40 it.

"Don't get up," I say, but Imre is already double-kissing me hello. "It's nice to see you," I add, and it's true. I always feel better when I'm singing and Imre's the kind of coach who knows when I need a compliment or a kick in the ass. *Shit.* I mean, bum.

"What's this?" he asks when he spies the IV pole that home care hasn't yet picked up, despite the fact that I finished treatment two weeks ago.

"Oh, it's nothing," I lie. "I had a relapse but I'm on the mend." Kind of true. I can lift my right leg off the ground for a few seconds—an improvement from the height of this attack, but not enough for the movement to feel reassuring.

"Relapse? What about the thing you had in Poland?" *What about it, indeed.* Another relapse so soon after CCSVI is a mind-fuck I can't begin to explain, not without saying the word *mind-fuck*.

"I'm okay, really. I had some trouble with my leg but it's getting better. Let's sing something!" Imre is making that face—the sad one with the wide eyes—that tells me he can't handle the truth, which I guess makes two of us.

"Okay. What do you want to start with? Anything to review?"

"I guess we should listen to my Easter performance. 'I Know That My Redeemer Liveth,'" I say, pulling up the recording on my computer. Post-performance game-tape analysis is always a little cringey but I'm thinking this one might feel more like torture. Imre looks back at the IV pole and raises an eyebrow.

"This Easter? As in two days ago?"

"Don't be too impressed. I didn't sing my best." *I didn't sing my best* is an understatement. I sound a little breathless and definitely unconvincing, like I don't know anything, let alone that my redeemer liveth. Go back to bed, Jesus. Sorry to wake you.

"The organ sounds great," Imre says, grasping for something good to focus on. "Who was playing?"

I don't take the bait. "I know I breathed all over the place, but at least it was in tune." Unfortunately only half this statement is true.

"You were still recovering; we don't need to hear the rest," Imre says three minutes into the six-minute aria.

"How bad is it?" I ask through gritted teeth.

"It's not as good as you can be. So what? Even on your worst day you're still a better singer than almost everyone else." I'm not out to trick the philistines into thinking I can sing, but I agree there's not a lot of value in this particular sample taken during exceptional, temporary circumstances.

"Thanks, Imre. Let's work on the recital rep." We start with "Am I Only Dreaming" because I know it so well I could sing it in my sleep, plus I find twentieth-century show tunes to be more forgiving than baroque coloratura.

"I think you need some water," Imre says after I struggle through the refrain. The high notes aren't coming easily and I'm getting flustered.

"What I need is some of that strong Hungarian *pálinka*," I joke, but Imre doesn't laugh.

"I'll bring you some if you make it through the next section without sneaking any breaths."

"Deal," I say. But it's a promise I can't keep.

"You need more time," Imre says after forty-five minutes of torturing the remainder of my rep. "We can cancel the recital."

"No," I say. I have a hard time believing there's anything productive about rest. I feel low-level anxiety if I'm not constantly working. Except for the five days I was on an elephant dose of steroids—which, at that volume, thin the voice and make practising counterproductive if not dangerous (assuming you also consider a little vocal strain a high-risk endeavour)—I never take a day off. I practise every day. Three hours. When I'm on vacation, I'll try to sneak in an hour before someone from the hotel complains. Singing is athletic. It's muscle memory. I can't afford to lose momentum. "We still have a few weeks," I say. "I can't cancel. I can't."

"We can always reschedule, do it in the summer," Imre offers. *Don't say* fuck *in front of Imre. Don't say* fuck *in front of Imre.* Rain checks aren't reliable when there's always more rain in the forecast. Perpetual motion keeps me tethered to what I have.

"Just think about it," Imre adds. "You're not where you were."

Ouch. Imre doesn't think I'm having an off day or even a bad week. He doesn't think my subpar singing is a blip or an anomaly. He thinks it's a regression. I feel so sad and overwhelmed because deep down I'm worried it's true. MS can eff up my legs, but I can't allow my voice to be affected by MS.

I'm close to panic. I'm not where I was but I have to get back there. "Imre, I can do this. I want you to push me."

"You're the boss," he says, shrugging.

That's right, MS motherfucker. *I'm* the boss.

THREE WEEKS LATER I feel beautiful standing next to the lacquered grand piano in my black gown with the peplum corset and long narrow skirt that has just a hint of a train. My hair's tied in a simple chignon and my cold hands are less cold than usual inside elbow-length vintage opera gloves—a gift from Tracy. They were her great-grandmother's.

Scanning the audience, I'm relieved to see a good-sized turnout. My whole family is here: my siblings; The Very Tall One's parents, the Svobodas; the core group of church choir cheerleaders; and a validating number of unfamiliar faces not driven by charity or obligation—people who presumably just want to hear some singing.

The audience is engaged and generous. Their applause justifies the encore I was going to sing anyway: "Am I Only Dreaming," a ballad from a past life, a song I first sang in high school. It was written for my voice by The Very Tall One, who is tragically no longer with us, after a sudden and unexpected cardiac death in 2004. He was twenty-seven.

> *Am I only dreaming? How I wish this were true . . .*
> *Soon I would be waking with a hundred things to do,*
> *No one knows the answers to the questions which I bear,*
> *Like am I only dreaming, or am I really here?*
> *Missions based on feelings, decisions left unclear,*
> *How to keep uncertainty from turning into fear?*

BACK AT OUR APARTMENT, The Banker beams with pride. "You fucking killed it," he says, because we speak the same language and Imre isn't within earshot. "I'm so proud of you," he adds, before kissing me goodnight.

Forty-five minutes later I'm still staring at the ceiling, but I don't curse the high that's keeping me up. Performance insomnia is a real phenomenon, a heady mix of relief, joy, pride and possibility. Today was a really good day and I'm happy to let it linger.

I worked hard to be ready for this recital, but the secret behind my high and my high notes was lowering just about everything else: lower shoes to keep me from teetering over in heels, lower sightlines thanks to the addition of a chair I wasn't too proud to use on stage. I even sang a couple of the most challenging tunes in a lower key.

I slayed some dragons today, but it wasn't a perfect performance. I'm still not where I was. Not even close. So why am I so euphoric?

I can't be mad at my A-flat when my recital raised five hundred dollars for the Wesley Centre. I can't dwell on vocal shortcuts when The Very Tall One's mother welled up with tears at the sound of her late son's song. I can't feel badly about breath control when my parents phone me two hours after gushing about my performance in person to gush about me some more.

But the real secret to my success feels like the very definition of a secret, because, as far as I know, nobody in the history of advice ever claimed without irony that the secret to success is lower expectations. I don't have to be great to be good, or even "good enough." I don't have to be the best to benefit from an experience.

MS makes you settle. One minute you're raging and resisting the unacceptable, the next minute you're clinging to any version of what's still possible, falling on your knees in gratitude for whatever the universe has left you. MS has been forcing me to be satisfied with church jobs and choral gigs since my mainstage dreams were first dashed a dozen years ago. And somehow I still feel so incredibly lucky that I get to do this amazing thing at all.

I know this bliss won't last, and if I'm being forced to figure out a new baseline, the cycle of existential bargaining will begin again. I promise to be happy with just this much. I will settle for the tiny sliver of singing I have and I will be grateful. Just as long as things don't get worse, as long as they stay the same.

Of course, nothing ever stays the same. Even settling is unsettling.

23 / Honourable Mention

A CHAIN-SMOKING, TEA-DRINKING INTELLECT, my maternal grandfather, Pappy, was a retired preacher and avid stamp collector who managed to turn me into a fellow philatelist by the age of ten, luring me into the hobby with gifts of what were basically princess stickers with a trade value.

I soon discovered that stamp collecting involved much more than hoarding treasures in a shoebox. Every good collection has a theme, and Pappy understood that my infatuation with the British monarchy was a gateway to collecting sticky scraps of government-issued memorabilia. I wasn't interested in rare finds, upside-down airplanes or misprints. I was into portraits of blue bloods in crowns and tiaras from as many countries as I could find. Pappy sourced the biggest, brightest, mint-condition postage stamps with smiling royals from around the world and I received them with delight. From heavy cardstock to display binders, mounts to soaking trays, I acquired an endless supply of tools and accessories to support my hobby. Aside from the stamps themselves, my most prized stamp-collecting paraphernalia were the bright gel pens I used to title my stamp display pages in my most carefully considered cursive.

Though I had zero talent for team sports, I wasn't a loner either. I was a social kid who, aside from reading, wasn't interested in pursuing reclusive hobbies. Fortunately, I was a natural ringleader, a yearbook shoo-in for *most likely to succeed at peer pressure*, and it didn't take much effort to convince my fifth-grade friends that stamp collecting was not just for old men and nerds: stamp collecting was cool.

Unlike baseball cards, which were good only for the stale rectangles of gum they were packaged with, stamp collecting encouraged all kinds of personal expression. Princes and princesses were my jam, but I assured my friends that they could build their own collections on anything from butterflies to horses to Disney characters. I sweetened the deal by sharing legends of rare finds that turned out to be worth millions, convincing my pals that a good collection could even be an investment, could maybe be worth something someday. And that's how Stamp Club was born.

Like any overachieving ten-year-old, I had a healthier-than-average relationship with the school principal, so it was easy to secure the library for our weekly Stamp Club meetings. My overly cautious mother, eager to co-sign an activity whose biggest risk was paper cuts, signed on as the parent volunteer.

Every Wednesday afternoon, my friends and I would gather to trade stamps, show off our latest acquisitions and take advantage of the library's books and encyclopedias to research the countries, figures and images that made up our collections. We'd savour deep drags of tropical fruit-scented markers, while the bitter glassine hinges polluted the taste of our after-school snacks. That a group of ten- and eleven-year-old girls would commit to such a dorky pastime was noteworthy enough that the local newspaper ran a story about our club with a colour photo and everything.

One day at Burlington's Imperial Coin & Stamp Co., the local shop where I spent my allowance on things like tongs, catalogues and one-dollar mystery bags, I saw a flyer advertising a Philately Expo, a full day event with vendors, booths, dealers, even a real-life auction. Best of all, there would be prizes for outstanding collections and anyone could enter. That stamp collecting—a sit-down sport that required brains—could be competitive added a whole new layer of excitement for me. And the Philately Expo appealed to me about as much as my school district's annual Battle of the Books tournament, which is to say, it appealed to me a lot.

The Philately Expo was held in the gym of a high school in Oakville, one town over. As my mom and I walked between rows of long tables searching for my submission amid the dozens on display, there wasn't another kid in sight. In a sea of black and white academic-looking exhibits, I was able to spot my colourful six-page spread two tables away.

That this wasn't a kids' event didn't deter me, though I was pretty bummed to discover that the "auction" turned out to be silent. I'd never heard of such a thing. I'd been expecting to see rich people with paddles angrily trying to outbid each other to the soundtrack of a fast-talking carny. I was hoping for a spectacle, not a yawn.

Finally it was time for the winning exhibits to be announced. Our collections were being judged on rarity, historical significance and presentation. My stamps were limited edition. Rare by definition. Issued in Niue, a small island in the South Pacific I'd never heard of before Pappy had gifted me the series of oversized glossy stamps I'd chosen to exhibit. I might have been excused for not having extensive knowledge of geography, but my parents had never heard of Niue either. A one-time British protectorate, the island is a self-governing territory in free association with New Zealand. Historically significant, my stamps commemorated the wedding of Prince Andrew to Sarah Ferguson, the red-headed duchess who I believed was cooler and even more beautiful than Princess Diana. As for presentation, my entry was in the bag. My collection was well formatted and full of facts. I was the only person who had thought to use glitter.

Third prize was called, then second, then first. Some guy, another guy, then some guy after that. Before I could register my heartbreak or outrage, a fourth category was called: Honourable Mention. The honouree was Ardra Shephard. *ME!* I was summoned to the stage, congratulated. I left with a swag bag of prizes, a one-hundred-dollar gift certificate to the Imperial Coin & Stamp and a fair amount of confusion.

I was proud of the advanced vocabulary my obsession with reading afforded me. *Silent auction* had been a hole in my knowledge that got filled with disappointment that day, but *honourable mention* was yet another new term to me. Sure, I had a drawer full of participation ribbons from track and field days, but those didn't come with any prizes. Nobody singled you out and called you to the stage. You and all the other uncoordinated awkwards were handed a participation ribbon with a Popsicle and the directive not to trip and fall on your way to the school bus. This didn't feel like that.

"WTF is honourable mention?" I asked my mother. (I didn't say "fuck," but it was implied.)

My mother scoffed. "Are you kidding me?" Her tone registered her own WTF feelings of disbelief that I could feel anything but honoured. "Honourable Mention is *better* than first place."

"How can anything be better than first place?" I asked.

"My dear," she said, "that award didn't *exist* until they saw your work.

Your pages were *so* good that they had to make a new award just for you. That's how special you are."

And I believed her.

My mom's ability to spin disappointment—to immediately pivot to silver linings—sometimes feels like blatant denial, protestant repression bordering on an unhealthy inability to process negative outcomes. But I can't deny the appeal of her unwavering belief in my own ability to kick ass. My parents' generation gets a lot of flack for creating an everyone-gets-a-ribbon culture, but maybe everyone *should* get a ribbon. Showing up is usually the hardest part.

When I was diagnosed, my dad told me that if anyone could handle MS, it was me. When people tell me they don't know how I do it, how I survive and even thrive despite MS, the answer, to me, lies in my inherent sense of self-worth. I'm not sure "anyone who doesn't think you're the best is stupid" is necessarily the best parenting strategy, but I always knew my parents thought I was smart and capable, talented and worthy.

When you are sick or disabled, the world tries to tell you a different story. The world tries to limit you, to make you small. I was taught to never hide my sparkle. Entitlement gets a bad rap, but feeling entitled to take up space, to contribute, to shine, to be celebrated has buffered me against the doubt and devaluing that can be inflicted on the chronically sick and disabled.

My parents' deluded faith in me has given me the deluded faith I've needed in myself.

24 / Take the Stares

IN 2010, MY BIG-CITY DREAMS came true when The Banker accepted a new job and we relocated to Toronto. Before moving into our new, much smaller apartment, we'd had a house-cooling party and invited our friends to leave with a lamp, an area rug, a wok or anything else we knew we wouldn't have room for. Both of our thrift shop–loving moms had shown up for our shindig half an hour early and giddily claimed most of our stuff, whether or not they'd needed it (they hadn't).

Our new Toronto pad is cozy, but it's all we need and less space to clean. Critically, we still have two bathrooms. Our loft ceilings are fourteen feet high and the building has a rooftop patio with a sunset view of Casa Loma, the city's famous Gothic Revival–style mansion. Our decor is part library, part brasserie, with a wall of floor-to-ceiling bookcases and an antique oak sliding ladder from a vineyard in Niagara. We asked everyone we invited to our house-warming party to bring a copy of their favourite book to add to our collection. The place doesn't have a killing room, but Torontonians seem to understand community living. We've been here for almost four years now; I sing all the time and no one has threatened to evict me.

One of the perks of our downtown location is the Baldwin Steps—a nineteenth-century stone staircase just a few minutes' walk from our apartment. Named after the Baldwin family (not that one), the 110 zigzagging steps are flanked by ancient trees. It's a beautiful, busy spot where Lululemon-clad runners compete for space with out-of-breath tourists who got off the subway at Dupont not realizing that the walk to Casa Loma is mostly vertical.

I spend the first few summers of Toronto life donning my own Lulus and dodging tourists, treating the steps like my personal outdoor gym. Using the railing as needed, left foot up, then the right, I take the stairs one at a time. I take the stares two or three at a time, but it didn't take long for the regulars—those runners who lap me before I've even reached the first landing—to start recognizing me. Their get-the-fuck-out-of-the-way glares have evolved into the occasional nod and split second of eye contact, signalling that they accept me as one of their own. Sort of. We're not friends, and that's fine. The only time I wanna hang out with a runner anyway is on carb-loading day. I don't want to hear about PBs, streaking or nipple chafing, ever, but it's nice to have my fitness journey acknowledged by these self-loathing psychos, to feel like I have just as much of a right to the Baldwin Steps as my health-seeking homies. Not like those annoying fucking tourists.

The strength-training goal I set for myself and have been working toward is ten flights: 1,100 stairs. Today, for the first time, I got there, albeit rabbit-and-tortoise style. Slow and steady. It took me over an hour. Even the most out-of-shape tourists were throwing shade as they passed me. The rabbits may have won the race, but I won the day. I'm proud of myself and my thighs, which are rock hard with muscle. My arms are beefy too, because I've been doing push-ups (push-aways?) against the railing in between flights. My Yankees cap, faded from the sun, is proof of how hard I've been working, of how many hours I've logged outside on these stairs. I take a big grinning selfie to commemorate my achievement and text it to The Banker: "1,100 steps! Aren't you proud of me!?"

Two days later I set out to crush my record. My new goal is ten and a quarter flights and not eleven, because crushing records when you have MS means setting realistic expectations. It's a hot day, though I don't think it's hotter than it has been, but by the time I get to five hundred steps, I feel myself fading. I now have a choice. I can chill out, go home, call it a day and start again tomorrow, or power through to prove to myself that I can still do at least ten flights, that I am as strong as I was two days ago, that MS isn't rearing its ugly fucking face.

In a plot twist that surprises even me, I cut myself some slack and go home. I take the rest of the day off and decide not to jump to conclusions.

A week later I'm wondering how the runners are doing and if anyone's noticed my absence. I haven't been back to the steps because I'm afraid of what I'll find out. I am so tired. The selfie I took a week ago already feels like a ghost of me.

This is the part of a potential relapse when I start testing every little thing, saying out loud what I observe and am afraid of until I'm sick of the sound of my own voice. Wondering if I'm just imagining a little numbness here, a little double vision there, though I almost never am.

Out in the real world it's more than just me noticing my sluggishness. The Banker and I are taking improv classes at The Second City (another perk of living in Toronto), and after class one night, The Banker and I walk with our troupe for drinks at a pub downtown. We've barely left the theatre when one of our classmates, Linda, asks, "Why are you walking like that?"

I have no answer. I don't want to "yes, and" her observation, plus I don't even know what *like that* means. Is it my lack of speed or does she see something else? Half a block later our group of twelve splits into two—the fast walkers keeping pace with Brian, our instructor, and the lollygaggers who either want to keep me company or who can't stand to hear about Brian's definitely terrible erotic Western novel one more time.

"What the fuck's the holdup?" Brian yells over his shoulder when he sees how far back we, the stragglers, are. What the fuck indeed.

Days later, a guy at the drugstore sees me leaning heavily on the makeup counter, and asks if I'm okay. There is nothing visibly wrong with me except for the fact that I'm wearing the wrinkled shirt I slept in, and so I feel the need to explain myself. "I have MS," I reveal, as if this explains a goddamn thing.

"Oh," he says. "Well, you'll be better by Christmas." It's not only random, it's an absurd prediction. This isn't a Hallmark movie. I'm not going to wake up healed on Christmas morning.

I don't have it in me to tell this guy about science. I should just say "thank you" and tell him I need to go get the tampons I came in for, but instead I start to cry, which turns out to be just as effective at ending our interaction. My miracle worker suddenly seems to understand he's out of his depth and backs out of our encounter without further attempts to soothe me.

The final straw, though, happens a few days later, an impossible two minutes from home.

"Hey, can you come pick me up?" I text The Banker, because I'm afraid I won't be able to keep it together if I call.

"Sure. Where are you?" he texts back. I'm up the street from our apartment. I can see the benches outside our building from my spot on the curb fifty feet away. I've been sitting on the sidewalk hoping to recover enough strength to walk the rest of the way, but now I'm not sure I can even stand up without help. I can't deny it any longer. This is a relapse. Almost a year to the day since my last one.

I want this time to be different—I want to handle an attack with grace—but I already blew that possibility when I cried in Shoppers Drug Mart.

I tell myself some trite twelve-hours-at-a-time bullshit I picked up I don't know where. I just need to focus on the twelve hours in front of me and the twelve hours after that. One day at a time, *rah rah, blah blah.* I believe it for all of twelve seconds, preferring to freak the fuck out. Twelve minutes later I take a deep breath and tell myself I know how to do this. I've done it before. I force myself to think about the book I'm reading or what I'll have for breakfast or what I'm going to wear to the opera next week. Outfit planning is my favourite distraction. Even if I feel like setting my workout clothes on fire.

I'm trying to outsmart my anxiety but my anxiety lives for moments like these. Why a relapse the moment I met my Baldwin Steps goal? Why did I have to wake the beast by bragging about how strong I was?

TB helps me into the apartment and I decide I need something to take the edge off before going to bed. I give myself props for not being a drug addict or an alcoholic—it would be so tempting not to feel any of this—then I chase a zopiclone with a double gin and tonic without the tonic. I'm trapped in a cycle of reason and hysteria until I exhaust myself like a toddler during a tantrum, but even exhaustion doesn't guarantee sleep.

Hysteria isn't sustainable and I am so fucking tired. *I know how to do this. I've done it before. I know how to do this. I've done it before. I know how to do this. I've done it before.* From the safety of my bed, I repeat this mantra in my mind, over and over again, waiting to believe it, or for the zopi-gin to kick in.

25 / Angry Dad

MY DAD IS AN EMOTIONAL GUY. Though he doesn't know it, he's listed in my phone as Angry Dad, an homage to Homer Simpson (this was from a time when *The Simpsons* was funny). Prone to catastrophizing and brooding, Angry Dad can, and frequently does, fly off the handle. He's not exactly known for his optimism or for keeping his chill. Certain stressors merit a degree of acrimony, but if the Hamilton Tiger-Cats lost their last CFL game, it's best to avoid him.

Angry Dad is capable of more emotions than anger, but there are no funny cartoons called Joyful Dad, though he is also prone to the condition. He delights in his grandchildren and looks forward to Christmas as much as they do. A lifelong learner, he's heavily involved in his community through acts of service and volunteering. He spends his downtime entertaining and writing detective novels.

I suspect I'm listed as some version of My Little Ardy in Angry Dad's own phone, or at least I would be if he knew how to customize his settings. Any version of *Ardy* might make it sound like I'm "Daddy's little girl," but Angry Dad has told me more than once that, in fact, he looks up to me. He says I'm his hero. To me, it's a ludicrous statement, but he defends the characterization, marvelling at how quickly I seem to bounce back from the depths of despair, wigging out one day, laughing the next. He wishes he could be more like that.

Angry Dad doesn't think he could handle what I handle, living with MS, and although I agree that there would be some bitching and complaining (and who could blame him?), I also believe that he would figure it out. Angry Dad doesn't give himself enough credit for what he has also survived: the things that made him angry in the first place.

Being called an inspiration or a hero often comes with the territory when living with a chronic illness or disability. I appreciate being recognized for being able to do hard shit, but it's impossible to handle MS with grace 100 percent of the time. Meanwhile, I, and many of my sick and disabled crew, bristle at being applauded for simply existing in our bodies. There's a fine line between pity and admiration. When the subtext of "I don't know how you do it" is "I'd probably kill myself if I were you," being told you're an inspiration lands less like a compliment and more like a slap in the face.

It's hard to argue with your dad, and even harder to change his mind. Angry Dad gets a pass for calling me his hero because he understands what people who feel sorry for me don't: that my life is hard, but that it's also pretty great too. Angry Dad believes these people would do well to replace their pity with envy.

Daddy's little girl or not, I'm a grown-up now, but even as an adult I still need my parents. Maybe that never goes away. I'm lucky I still have them. Although I can count on my mom to champion and cheerlead, to gossip and talk fashion, Angry Dad's superpower revealed itself the first time I had a truly epic MS meltdown. And at every meltdown since. When I am utterly beside myself, my dad listens and consoles. Without trying to fix it, he sits with me in my torment in a way that few others can. I never feel like I've given him more than he can handle. He somehow knows the exact moment when I am ready to be reminded of who I am. Handling my meltdowns is Angry Dad at his best.

I can count on one hand the number of times I have been so out of control that I've needed to take advantage of this special-occasion service. I don't cry wolf unless a wolf is in the house.

It's time to call my dad.

26 / H Is for Hope

DR. POKER FACE TELLS ME there are only three tiny new lesions on my latest MRI. The words *only* and *tiny* are supposed to encourage me to process my results as good news, I guess, because I live in a world where only a little bit of additional brain damage is something I'm supposed to celebrate, or at least be grateful for.

The three new polka dots that decorate my brain aren't the whole picture anyway. My brain's lesion load has historically been relatively light. Most of my MS lives on my cervical spine, where even tiny lesions can cause massive problems. *Why aren't we scanning my spinal cord?* is a question I didn't know I was supposed to be asking.

New lesions or not, I can feel myself getting weaker, slower, insidiously slipping away from my once familiar body. *I'm getting worse and I'd prefer to freak out about it, thanks.*

"I'm afraid I'm going to need a wheelchair," I say, because it's true: it's my biggest fear (so far) and I need to be sure that the guy in charge of looking after me understands.

"I know," says Dr. Poker Face, true to his matter-of-fact self.

"There has to be something else we can do!"

Says who? Not logic. Not science. I have no inherent right to be healed of this disease.

Dr. Poker Face takes a beat.

"I'll refer you to Ottawa, if you're still interested in stem cells," he says, like it's no big deal, but my eyes bug out of my head.

"SERIOUSLY?" My heart skips a beat and I make him say it again. I've been asking to participate in the Canadian HSCT trials since 2001.

"HSCT is a complex high-risk procedure," he reminds me.

Yeah, I know. The *H* in HSCT stands for *hematopoietic*, a word so complex it's literally unpronounceable. To recap: a hematopoietic stem cell transplant means wiping out your immune system with a serious amount of chemo and then resetting it with your own pre-harvested stem cells. It's an immune-system reboot to trick your body into forgetting that it wants to destroy you. The risks include infection, organ damage, infertility, cancer, respiratory issues, cardiovascular problems, probably herpes—basically a long list of shit that ends with "you're not likely to die, but you could," and I'm ready to roll the dice on all of it. Sign me up, because you know what else is risky? Fucking out-of-control MS.

"I'll send your file to Ottawa, and it will be up to them to decide if you're a suitable candidate."

Dr. Poker Face's final comment pushes my bugged-out eyeballs back into my head as I realize HSCT is not yet a done deal: I will be on a wait-list until who knows when, and I still have to convince yet another lab coat that I'm a good fit for this procedure I'm so desperate to have. Nonetheless, I leave the appointment feeling buoyant. I'm not quite ready to open myself up to feeling hopeful, but I am energized, excited. I have a plan.

Over the next few weeks, waiting for my consultation to be scheduled causes me PMS-on-Adderall-level mood swings. I spend hours researching the procedure, bursting into tears at least once a day, reading about miraculous recoveries as well as worst-case scenarios and everything in between. I get in touch with a woman who credits the procedure with saving her life. I don't have the courage to ask her why she's now crowdfunding a wheelchair if HSCT worked so well. I am legitimately confused. I talk to another patient who had severe complications and needed a lung transplant. He survived and says his MS is now basically a non-issue. A lung transplant is no joke, but it's reassuring to see the high level of attention and care patients are getting in Ottawa. There are enough success stories to reinforce my belief that HSCT is the only way to turn my MS around.

27 / Pros and Cons

"PROS AND CONS," I say, curling up on the couch to face The Banker, before taking a haul off a goblet of wine so big I need two hands to hold it. It's Family Meeting time, and there's only one item on the agenda, but it's a big one. We should probably be sitting at a proper table, wearing spectacles and looking serious; maybe there's a moderator or even a stenographer. Instead, I'm in pyjamas, hoping that low lighting and a slight buzz will make this attempt at domestic democracy feel incidental or even benign. Family Meetings are supposed to be about where to vacation or what to do about Uncle Vic, not highly consequential determinations of how much my well-being is worth in literal dollars. And not even regular dollars, but expensive-ass American ones.

"What's on your list?" I ask.

Democracy isn't perfect, and admittedly our marriage is more of a monarchy anyway—an Ardra-archy, if you will. It's a mutually beneficial, if unspoken arrangement *chez nous*. The Banker is slow to embrace change or make decisions and I am a woman of action. I can be impulsive, and I'm rarely inert. Okay, that last part is a lie. I'm what doctors call "sedentary," the poster girl for "sitting is the new smoking," but that doesn't mean I don't make shit happen. I don't need a month of recon to decide what car to buy, what colour to paint the walls or whether or not we should have Uncle Vic for dinner (we should not). Ardra-archy isn't perfect, but the consequences are mostly limited to the occasional bout of decision fatigue and enduring The Banker's passive-aggressive observations about how much I spent on the latest luxury dog bed.

Even so, some decisions cannot be made unilaterally and this is one of them. Suddenly I have a chance to have HSCT in Chicago immediately, at our own expense, or I can continue to wait indefinitely for my referral to Ottawa, with no guarantee I'll be treated. Sounds like a no-brainer for my brain damage, but brain damage is notoriously complicated.

"Pros: you might get better," The Banker opens. Okay, a little obvious, but we're just getting started, so I let it slide and take another haul of my Montepulciano.

"Pros: Chicago is faster, and there's less time for me to have another relapse," I say.

"Pros: Chicago's protocol is safer," he adds.

"Because their protocol is less aggressive, so that's actually a con," I counter.

"*Slightly* less aggressive," he says, as if there's room for "slightly" when we're discussing degrees of disability. "Pros: If Chicago could get you in by February, we wouldn't have to go to Darrel's stag and doe."

"That is a compelling point. Let's move that to the top of the list."

"Pros: We could visit Wrigley Field, try deep-dish pizza . . ."

"Those sound like cons to me. Next."

"Cons: Who will look after the dog?" TB's dodging the subject, trying to buy time before getting to what this is really about.

"Figuring out who gets to hang with Rihga isn't a con, it's an administrative detail," I say. "Cons: I'll be isolated from everyone for months."

"That would be true in Ottawa too." He's right. We're losing the plot. I've already considered these factors. It's not about whether or not I should have the procedure, but where.

"Cons: What if I get treated in the US and a Canadian doctor refuses to give me follow-up care?"

"Can they do that?"

"I think so, yeah."

"I think I've run out of pros." He pauses, noticing my raised eyebrow and refusal to fill the ensuing silence. "But Chicago is a bird in the hand and Ottawa is—"

"Free," I say, finishing his sentence, and saying what he won't. Because if cost weren't a factor, I'd already be in Chicago getting ready to burn my immune system to the ground. Cost is the uncomfortable bottom line.

"We should go to Chicago," he says, but I'm not convinced he believes it. "We could do a fundraiser," he adds, in an attempt to convince me that he's serious, but I hear only his unspoken anxiety about just how much this will cost.

"Babe, we do not hang out with the kind of people who can drop a hundred Gs at a bake sale."

"Two hundred."

"What?"

"We'd need closer to two hundred Gs," he clarifies.

"So in your mind we fundraise the whole thing? A garage sale? And a GoFundMe?" I can't help it, but my tone is bordering on bitchy. I take a deep breath and another sip of wine, because I don't want this Family Meeting to dissolve into an argument. I need us to be productive so we don't ever have to have this conversation again.

"We'll figure it out. We'll find a way," he says. He's trying to sound like he means it.

"But what if we put all our resources behind this and I still get sicker?"

"You won't."

"I might."

"We'd handle it."

"How do you know?"

"How do you not? We always handle it." His eyes are wide, like he's trying to force his conviction into my brain. It's a fair point.

"I don't want to fundraise or ask anyone for money. It's too much pressure to produce a return on everyone's investment."

"Then we'll talk to the bank, cash in our savings, take out a loan," he says, like it's easy. Like his love language isn't registered retirement savings vehicles, safety nets and living well within our means.

"I don't want you to resent me if we sell the condo, wipe out our savings, blow it all up and I don't get better."

He bristles at the implication. "I would never resent you! Never!" To his credit, I believe he believes this.

"We would be sacrificing our whole lifestyle. I don't want us to have to give up travelling." How can I expect The Banker to be possessed of some monk-like lack of resentment when I myself would resent what we would be giving up?

"I can't believe you would put a price on your life," he says. I can't believe it either. I am not the financially responsible one in this relationship. But if the tables were turned, I know we wouldn't be having this conversation.

The Banker always puts me first. We live in the city that was my first choice, in a building that accommodates my accessibility needs. He rearranges his work schedule to take me to appointments so that I don't have to take transit. He suffers through extremes of indoor climate control, has watched every episode of *Gilmore Girls* and yields the banquette at every bistro. The Banker isn't capable of making a decision that's best for us, only what's best for me.

Being treated like a queen sounds good on paper, and yes, it is amazing to be loved and looked after to this degree. I try to remind myself that when one person has MS, the whole house has MS, that MS is a team sport; we just have different positions managing it. The Banker is always willing to take one for the team, but even with his unwavering support, MS still feels like my problem—like I am the problem to be solved.

I have years of experience running the numbers, doing the math on what percentage of our resources is reasonable to spend on my medications, vitamins, supplements, special diets, physiotherapy, mobility aids, catheters, leg braces, pressure-sore pillows, massage therapy, experimental treatments and more. I am a one-woman industry and it's hard to say how much of a difference any of these interventions has made—my MS keeps getting worse. A better bookkeeper could tell you how much I've already cost us. In dollars, in time, in experiences. It's easy to feel like I take more than I give, when what's mine is yours and what's yours is . . . my medical expenses.

I stopped believing in things turning out as they're meant to a long time ago. I'm a fan of autonomy, agency and, let's face it, control. I'm not a Jesus-take-the-wheel kind of girl, and I'm not a gambler either. I'm willing to risk my life for a chance to be better, but not my life *and* our livelihood.

"Let's put our faith in Ottawa," I say, toning down my Ardra-archal tone and choosing a team-captain approach instead. Making monumental decisions that impact more than just me is one of the invisible symptoms of MS; it's one of the burdens. Chicago doesn't feel like what's best for the whole, but it's nice to know that The Banker would have put on his game face and rallied for me if I'd asked him.

AT MY THIRTY-EIGHTH birthday dinner, once my siblings have left, TB and I sit down with my parents and I explain the procedure I'm after. My voice breaks when I tell them that for the first time I'm allowing myself to consider a future that doesn't involve a wheelchair. I briefly burst into tears, then quickly get a hold of myself. I continue to explain the facts—the chemo, the isolation, the early menopause—while The Banker sits next to me with his hand on my knee. What I really need them to understand is that if something terrible should happen, I would stand by my decision. I need them to know that I accept and am comfortable with the risks. Jim and Norma listen quietly without interrupting (me or each other), a rare and off-brand reaction, and when I'm done talking, they both affirm that they are on board without hesitation. Once again, my dad tells me that I'm his hero, but I'm only trying to save myself. Whether or not I will have the option is up to someone else.

28 / Hair Today, Gone Tomorrow

"I'M THINKING OF GOING BLACK," I say, but the truth is, I've already decided.

"*Black*, black?" Jaz asks with a reasonable amount of skepticism. "It's just that red suits you so much."

My pale skin, green eyes and freckles mean I could almost pass for a natural redhead. Feisty, with a higher-than-average tolerance for pain and a lower-than-average tolerance for bullshit, my temperament backs up the stereotypes. Even my name means "ardent," which is basically a synonym for *fiery*. A certain kind of woman chooses to be a redhead and it's a choice I've been making since I was thirteen, spending my babysitting money at The Body Shop on ten-dollar packages of henna until I could afford proper salon visits. Red is a state of mind. And that's the problem. I don't feel like myself.

I'm not trying to go goth. I just need something different, something dramatic. I want out of this body, and a change of hair colour seems more reasonable than escaping through drugs or alcohol.

"If you don't like it, it will be too hard to undo," Jaz tries to reason. I spy her making eye contact with one of her colleagues, who chimes in to back her up.

"You're so fair, and black looks . . . kinda angry?" This is a proper salon. They don't do emo here. Still, I don't give in.

"Liv Tyler, Julianna Margulies, Angelina Jolie . . . they're all pale with dark hair," I reason, listing my late-1990s/early-aughts icons without mentioning the true pale icons I resemble: Malfoy, Casper and the Michelin Man. I affectionately think of my legs as my personal solar panels, but one time, when we were on a beach vacation, a stranger told The Banker that I looked like a daywalker in my bikini. The number-one comment I get from online trolls is "get a tan."

"Maybe we could try a dark brown instead of jet black? Something with warm undertones?" Jaz is practically pleading.

"Fine," I concede, if only because I'm sad (but I'm not so sad that I would consider an at-home dye job). "Let's do dark brown, but I want extensions too."

Four hours later my red bob has been replaced by rolling waves of chestnut-coloured boob-length hair. I move my head from side to side, appreciating my hair's unfamiliar volume and foreign texture (it's literally from India). I have a mild headache from the metal beads that sit close to my scalp, securing my luscious new locks to the baby-fine hair I was born with.

There's nothing new about changing your hair as catharsis. My body might be out of control, but I'm still in charge of my hair. It hardly matters that it doesn't look good—I don't look like me anymore, and that's the point.

Two weeks later, I haven't fully adjusted to the extreme amount of conditioner my new look demands, but I have come up with an idea for a blockbuster crime novel about a woman who is wrongfully convicted of a gruesome murder based on DNA testing of hair that turns out to be extensions. Meanwhile, my new 'do hasn't solved my old problems, but it has created some new ones, like clogged drains. It's impossible to rinse all the shampoo out of more hair than I've had in a lifetime and I tell myself getting most of the suds out is good enough. In a plot twist I didn't see coming, my hair ends up controlling me after all.

A few days after I get the extensions, sudden hope arrives when Ottawa calls and offers me the HSCT consult. I feel like I've won the lottery and accept their next available appointment.

The Banker and I make the drive to Ottawa, four hundred kilometres from home. I feel like I hit the jackpot, but I still have to answer the skill-testing question in order to collect my prize. The stakes are high and the question I've got one shot at answering is: Why should I be one of the one or two patients chosen each year to receive this life-changing treatment?

I normally don't bring The Banker to my medical appointments, but if I'm offered HSCT, it won't be something I can do alone. He needs to know what to expect and how to support me. Plus, I'm nervous as hell; this is a really big deal and I'm grateful for the Team Ardra energy his presence provides.

I'm handed a clipboard and a stack of paperwork in the waiting room of the Ottawa Hospital MS Clinic—all standard stuff except for the one-page document that asks about the last time I drove a car. I get it. Nobody wants the optic-neuritis-ed among us to be operating heavy machinery. I haven't done anything wrong—I haven't driven in fourteen years—but being asked to put that fact in writing makes me defensive. It doesn't help that I actually feel like I'm trying to get away with something here, pleading my case for a procedure that feels like my only hope. The passive-aggressive paperwork is another reminder that I'm not the one who's in charge.

The doctor–patient power dynamic is further reinforced when the next thing I'm asked to do is step on a scale. A weigh-in has never been part of my previous neuro exams. It's true that excessive weight can worsen MS symptoms, but "just lose weight" is a dismissive refrain that wreaks of blaming and shaming people for their disease. Neuro appointments are stressful enough, especially for women wanting invisible symptoms to be taken seriously. Seems to me that the weigh-in could wait until after a supportive environment has been established. (Just a thought.)

Finally, we meet the doctor in charge of my fate. Bald, in a white lab coat and glasses, he looks like Dr. Bunsen Honeydew from *The Muppets*—a look that's hard to reconcile with his I-know-I'm-the-shit energy. This man is no puppet. I can't be mad at his vibe. He is kind of a big deal in the MS world. And, except for this precise moment, I usually carry myself like I know I'm the shit too. Plus, if someone's gonna explode my immune system, I'd like them to have a metric fuck-tonne of confidence.

The mood is intense as Dr. Muppet examines me. The Banker has been tasked with keeping quiet and taking notes. Time is precious, and I know he will have a long list of questions, but I don't want him asking any of them—at least not at this initial appointment. I don't want TB giving the impression we have any doubts.

Dr. Muppet talks quickly. He talks over me, and he can be brusque. I'm trying to retain not just the words he's saying but the tone of the room, and the energy of the nurse, who is quiet but focused. I want to absorb all the details that contribute to this experience, because I am hyper-aware that even within the scope of a medically exceptional life, none of this is routine. I live with extraordinary circumstances and today could be the beginning of a journey I will want to remember in detail.

"You use a catheter and you have a history of UTIs," Dr. Muppet says. "That's a concern." My heart quickens at the first suggestion that I might not be a suitable candidate for immune-system ablation.

"Surely everyone with MS who has HSCT has a bladder problem? This must be a risk we can mitigate," I protest. Dr. Muppet is already moving on to his next talking points.

"This is chemo—you could die." *Yeah, I fucking know.*

"Most of the patients we treat have an EDSS of six. Yours is only 4.5, and even then, it's only that high because of your vision and bladder."

Wait, am I too sick or not sick enough? EDSS—the Expanded Disability Severity Scale—is bullshit anyway. EDSS is skewed to recognize mobility without much consideration for the many ways in which MS can be disabling.

"My legs seem strong now because I've just spent an hour sitting in the waiting room. If I had to walk around the block a couple of times, I'd come back limping," I say, trying to prove I warrant treatment. "My feet are constantly blue and so cold; it makes it hard to sleep."

"Is that true?" he asks The Banker, instead of me. TB verifies my claim.

"Wait a few years and menopause will take care of that," Dr. Muppet says, chuckling. I can't tell which one of us this comment is meant for, but I can see which way this appointment is going and I don't like it.

"When do you go back to Toronto?" he asks as my examination starts to wrap up.

"We're driving home tomorrow."

"Book her an MRI and a lumbar puncture for tomorrow morning, first thing," Dr. Muppet tells his nurse, like this is a normal request and not an outrageous demand. "You can drive home after that," he adds, definitely talking to The Banker. It's already close to 5 p.m., and as far as I know, next-day MRIs are for A-list professional athletes and visiting popes, should they need one: V-I-fucking-P, and next to impossible to get. When the nurse comes back fifteen minutes later saying that she bumped an in-patient and got both appointments booked, I try not to let my eyes pop out of my head. That Dr. Muppet gets what Dr. Muppet wants makes his personality more palatable. At least in this instance.

"Great!" I say, though what I'm actually thinking is, *Shit*. I was not expecting to need an MRI on such short notice. I run my fingers through my long wild hair, finally regretting my salon choices, but not for the reason Jaz predicted. You can't have any metal on or in your body during an MRI. Instead of voicing my concerns that an MRI with metal beaded extensions would turn me into a human fragmentation bomb, I slap on a smile and say, "See you in the morning." I don't want to jeopardize my chance at HSCT. It's fine. I've got fourteen hours to figure it out, and I am a problem-solver.

"That was exhausting. I'm starving. What do you feel like for dinner?" TB asks in the car as we're leaving the hospital.

"We can't eat yet. There's a Canadian Tire seven minutes away," I say, checking my phone. "It closes in fifteen minutes." There are no after-hours emergency hair salons in Ottawa, so Canada's favourite hardware store will have to suffice. "I need you to run in and pick up a pair of pliers. The smallest ones you can find."

"For what?!" The Banker asks with genuine bewilderment at what is an unexpected Team Ardra request.

An hour later I'm eating pizza on the hotel bed while The Banker bends over me with a new pair of pliers.

"Sheppy, I don't feel good about this. What if I cut out clumps of your hair?"

"Slow and gentle. You're just loosening the beads. Let's watch the YouTube tutorial again." I'm nervous too, but I don't dare admit it. I consider incentivizing him by telling him how much money we're saving with this DIY, but that would mean copping to how much I've already wasted on my latest reinvention.

The first pieces come out with minimal swearing and moderate amounts of my original hair. Only once does any of it graze the pizza.

"You really couldn't have had this MRI in Toronto?"

"It's a good sign," I say. Dr. Muppet means business.

THE NEXT MORNING I arrive at my ongoing audition to be the clinic's next favourite patient looking like I've already started chemo. I keep what's left of my patchy 'do tucked into my winter hat all day and try not to think about the hotel housekeeper's reaction to finding a garbage can full of hair. If Dr. Muppet notices my dramatic make-under, he doesn't mention it.

"This is Dr. Muhammad, the intern who will be doing your lumbar puncture. I'll be back after I've looked at your MRI." A lumbar puncture (LP) is a medical procedure used to collect a sample of cerebrospinal fluid (CSF). LPs can help diagnose MS and I've never had one because when Dr. Poker Face mentioned "lumbar puncture" at the time of my diagnosis, my mom said, "Oh no. She's not having a spinal tap." And that was that.

But proving I can handle HSCT means showing off my plucky I-can-do-hard-things persona at every opportunity. I agree to give an extra sample because this is a research hospital. *Mi spinal fluid es su spinal fluid. Help yourself. Take as much as you need! You want to let a student put a four-inch needle directly in my spine? Sure! What could go wrong?*

"You're lucky you're so small," the intern tells me with some excitement. "We have to go pretty deep on bigger people."

"Can I see the needle you'll be using?" I ask, doubling down on my bravado. It's fucking enormous. *Bring it on.*

"This is the needle we use on the larger ones," he says, holding an even bigger tool that looks like it should be used on a horse or in a cartoon.

At this point The Banker is asked to leave. It's a good call. He looks like he wants to pass out.

"The first needle will feel like dental freezing." It's hard to imagine the sensation of dental freezing in my back but that's exactly what it's like. It takes a long time to collect my CSF and I'm chatty and brave, even though I wish I'd been sedated.

"So, what exactly does cerebrospinal fluid do?" I ask, like I don't already know.

"CSF surrounds the brain and spinal cord, cushioning the central nervous system in a protective barrier. The liquid is clear, but it takes a while to get a sample because it has the consistency of maple syrup." It's the most Canadian statement I have ever heard. I'm being tapped like a tree.

When the procedure is over, I'm told to lie flat for at least an hour. I can't even have a pillow. Until the wound closes up, I'm at risk of Ardra syrup leaking throughout my body.

"If the puncture doesn't seal, it will be the worst headache of your life," the intern warns me. By sometime tomorrow evening I will learn that "worst headache of my life" is a massive understatement. In the meantime, I lie flat as a pancake.

"THERE ARE NO SIGNS of PML on your MRI," Dr. Muppet says. That's good, I think, though I wasn't actually worried about progressive multifocal leukoencephalopathy. PML is something that needs to be ruled out before starting immune-suppressing treatment. "There are no enhancing MS lesions either; your MRI is stable." This is also good, but maybe not? His voice has a "you'd better sit down" quality, but I'm already lying down and I can't read his expression.

"I want you to try alemtuzumab. It's just been licensed for MS. It's an immunotherapy that, like HSCT, resets the immune system, but with fewer risks." *Yeah,* I think to myself. *I know all about it.*

But Dr. Muppet gets what Dr. Muppet wants and suddenly alemtuzumab feels like a foregone conclusion. Unfortunately, I've been forced into submission by the puncture wound in my spine. It's an inconvenient time to panic.

"I don't want safer, I want effective. I want the Mack truck of treatments to obliterate this disease," I plead to the fluorescent light on the ceiling.

"Think of alemtuzumab as HSCT Lite," Dr. Muppet continues as if this is a selling feature. Calling alemtuzumab HSCT Lite just adds insult to injury. As if "lite" ever yielded anything less than inferior. I don't want the imitation-cheese version of MS treatments.

"And what if alemtuzumab doesn't work?" I feel defeated. I'm out of my depth.

"Then we'll give you HSCT." It seems like a fair compromise, but treatment with alemtuzumab takes two years. HSCT is most effective early in the disease. The longer I have MS, the less likely I am to get HSCT. I'm running out of time. I don't know what I can say to convey my urgency.

"I'm afraid I'm going to be in a wheelchair." It's the same thing I told Dr. Poker Face. In contrast to Dr. Poker Face's empathetic if impotent reply, Dr. Muppet gives me the answer I need to hear.

"I won't let that happen," he says. It's a balls-out statement that reeks of irresponsibility and a God complex. I know it's an empty promise, but logical me has left the building. I want to believe it so bad. I didn't win the HSCT lottery. Alemtuzumab is my consolation prize. I don't have the luxury of dwelling on my own disappointment. The only real choice I have is to be devastated at being denied full-fat HSCT or get on board with HSCT Lite.

On his way out of the room, Dr. Muppet gives my foot a squeeze, and more than his outsized confidence, it's this sign of humanity that reassures me that plan B might work out.

"You heard what he said, right?" I ask the nurse after he leaves. "You heard him say that if this drug fails, he will give me HSCT?" I sound desperate and probably pathetic. I'm not looking for clarification; I know exactly what was said. I ask the nurse to repeat it because I want a witness.

"Yes," she confirms in what I must know, on some level, is a useless testimony. She has no more power here than I do. That I even asked the question means I don't fully trust this situation.

I didn't get what I came for, but I can't afford to feel defeated. In an act of self-preservation, I control the only thing I can, which is my perspective. I tell myself we're leaving Ottawa with a positive outcome, a solid plan and world-class care, but The Banker's not convinced. He's still Team Ardra, and he can't hide his disappointment.

29 | *Tripping on Air*

IT'S BEEN MORE THAN fourteen years since my MS diagnosis, and six months since I last sang in public. Since I sang at all. We don't always know when we're doing something for the last time and I can't pinpoint the moment I knew I was no longer a singer. Worse still, I don't yet know who I will be next.

The joy I got from singing eroded slowly, almost imperceptibly. When new arias felt especially difficult, I thought I just needed to work harder. I didn't understand that MS was impacting my breath, making my voice weaker and my high notes harder to reach, until I started needing extended breaks during coaching sessions and found myself having to sit on a chair through entire lessons. I stopped looking for improvements in my repertoire and became desperate to preserve the skills I'd worked so hard to cultivate, but my lowered expectations were outpaced by my decline.

If I can't be a singer, I have to be something else. I need a sense of purpose or I will lose my mind. This isn't my first attempt to reinvent. I do what has worked before and make an updated list of things I like or am good at: languages, art, travel, food, fashion, relationships. I don't overthink it and keep the pen moving, adding baking, talking, cheese, gossip and having a disease.

This is a brainstorm, so technically there are no wrong answers, but I'm not actually good at baking. I'm not even sure I enjoy it—I just like having muffins around.

Cheese is on the list as if cheese were a verb. Is "cheese whisperer" a thing? I like eating cheese, overspending on cheese, putting cheese labels in a stinky cheese diary with notes about flavour, consistency and odour, but I don't make cheese, or sell it.

Maybe I'll start a book club. Of course, a book club is only profitable if your name is Oprah or Reese Witherspoon. Plus, a book club feels like a direct path to a drinking problem.

I'm pretty good at languages. I speak French and watched *Narcos* without the subtitles, an educational experience that filled in the vocabulary gaps that Rosetta Stone didn't cover, but being able to speak Drug Cartel doesn't exactly qualify me to be a translator, or even a tutor.

I consider my affection for gossip, dissecting relationship dynamics and being self-analytical. I like thinking, figuring shit out. Problem-solving. Not math problems, unless you count mixing fabric prints, or figuring out hemline-to-bare-leg ratios, which, technically, I guess is math. Maybe we're getting somewhere.

Unlike my love for cheese, I don't like having a disease, but I am legitimately good at it, even if I've been in the cheese game for twice as many years as I've had MS. (I didn't say I was Terry Wahls. I'm good at *having* MS, not *curing* it.) Fourteen years equals more than 122,000 hours of practice, which, according to Malcolm Gladwell, means I could be a world-class disease-having expert more than twelve times over. And yeah, sleep hours count in this equation, because bladder urgency, spasticity and nerve pain don't clock out at bedtime.

One of my more appealing ideas is Old Lady Biographer, a job I just invented where families hire me to conduct in-depth interviews with their elderly matriarchs and then write their biographies—not for publication, but to have a family history. I like writing and storytelling, so OLB has potential, but I'm in an extended period of self-absorption right now and realize I would rather tell stories about *me*.

Which leaves the itchiest option of all: blogger. I swore I'd never write a blog. Self-indulgent, narcissistic—bloggers are the worst (at this point in time, podcasting has yet to fully take off). I have to admit, though, that blogging has the potential to tick a lot of my raison d'être boxes. The blogosphere is already oversaturated with art, travel and fashion content, and I'm pretty sure nobody wants to read more than a sentence about why you should save your cheese rinds for making soup. When considering my potential niche, the only topic that makes sense is MS. I could be my own Old Lady Autobiographer.

I never wanted to be a spokesperson for a crappy disease I didn't sign up for, but somebody has to take the mic. When it comes to MS, in 2015, the information superhighway doesn't have a lot of super information. The basic facts are there, but the kind of practical inside scoop I once needed, and still need, is missing. Sorry, Montel, Squiggy and Richard Cohen, but in a disease that predominantly affects young women, your stories—all written from a male patient's perspective—haven't been much help to me. (Marc Stecker's fantastic science-y blog, *Wheelchair Kamikaze*, which makes sense of medical research and new treatments, notwithstanding.)

My advanced degree in life's hard knocks qualifies me to talk about the skills I've learned and the information I wish someone had shared with me. If I were to write a blog, it would be filled with the life hacks you need to know that no one tells you. I could talk about the pain of giving up high heels in a post I might call "Shoe-icide." I could write catchy listicles with advice on what to pack for a day at Spa-udemdrol. I would demystify and destigmatize the miracle that is Cathy. My blog would be pink and pretty and fun. Not because MS is pink and pretty and fun, but because I am.

I spend as much time thinking about what my blog could be as I do thinking about what it must not be. I refuse to be the tragic main character of my own story (though, rest assured, I am the main character). I'm not interested in writing stories to remind the masses that their own lives could be worse. No pity, but no bullshit either.

I'm sick of hearing things like "you have nothing if you don't have your health." The internet is heavy on the promise that MS doesn't have to stop you, that MS shouldn't define you. If I had a blog, it would have the courage to acknowledge that MS stops me all the time—it literally stops me every day. That doesn't mean I'm failing at having a disease. Or at life. MS stops me. It's not my fault. And like Larry David says, "Some people are nothing even *with* their health."

Saying "MS doesn't define me" lives in the realm of "methinks the lady doth protest too much." Why would I feel the need to voice opposition to that which is benign? If I started insisting that my freckles don't define me, it might be safe to assume that my freckles were having some kind of outsized influence on how I see myself.

I didn't choose my freckles any more than I chose to have MS, but they both contribute to my identity. You say "sun damage" and I say "angel kisses." I'll never think of MS as charming, but I do get to decide exactly how I perceive it.

As I consider my options, I realize that a blog could be a way for me to push back against the assumptions and misconceptions about what it means to live with MS. A blog could help me push back against the idea that allowing MS to be part of my identity (like I have a choice!) is something to be ashamed of.

Nora Ephron once said, "When you slip on a banana peel, people laugh at you. But when you tell people you slipped on a banana peel, it's your laugh—so you become the hero rather than the victim of the joke." Replace "slip on a banana peel" with "pee your pants at the mall" and that's why I want to write about MS. It's my story and I control the version. Nobody need whisper about the tragedy that is my life, because I went ahead and decided it's a rom-com instead.

My blog will need a catchy title. *Life Lesions* is a contender. *Multiple Shit-osis* feels a bit too negative, *SclerosterCoaster* is kind of a mouthful. In the end, I decide to call my blog *Tripping on Air: My Trip through Life with MS*. I can't imagine writing will bring me the kind of joy that singing once did, but my hope is that it will give me a renewed sense of purpose. Maybe writing about MS will help me find some meaning in this shit show; maybe my wisdom won't feel like wasted knowledge. I want *Tripping on Air* to tell the whole truth: MS is hard. Here's what you can do about it.

30 / Disability Awareness

I THINK I'M THE LAST TO KNOW, but today was the first day I realized I no longer have an invisible illness, and it landed like an epiphany. Not one of the good epiphanies either, like when I discovered dry shampoo. More like one of the inconvenient End Times ones from the Book of Revelation.

It's true that lately I've been hearing a lot more "what's wrong with your legs?" comments than "you look so good," and I guess if I'd thought about it, I would've realized I've been straddling the blurry line between "invisible illness" and "visibly disabled" for a while now. Progression doesn't announce itself with a bang (although there are a considerable number of falls); it comes and goes and comes and goes and comes, and eventually it just stops going.

Meanwhile, I've been trading breast self-exams for neuro self-exams and feeling gaslit by my body. (Just kidding, I never do breast exams.) But I do test my legs. All the time. I'm not sure when I had to start measuring the total number of individual stairs I can climb instead of counting by flights, or when I switched to sussing out how long I can walk on the treadmill before my foot starts kicking the belt. My little tests, degrading in difficulty (along with my morale and standards). It would be easier to put my pants on sitting down, but I do it standing just to make sure I still can. My research suggests progression is lurking, but, until today, I had yet to conclude that my illness is no longer invisible.

My disability awakening happened on a Sunday, just outside of Toronto, in the closest approximation of a church I've been to lately. Weekends are for brunch and bakery crawls and that's how The Banker and I ended up in Oakville, forty minutes west of Toronto (five and a half hours if there's traffic), at Monastery Bakery.

I'm serious about bakeries. I'm always on the hunt for the perfect pastry shop with an old-school hanging doorbell and a Juliette Binoche–type proprietor who can tell just by looking that some combination of lavender, bergamot and butter will heal all my past and future heartbreak, a place where I can ooh and aah over delicate raspberry-topped confections that look too pretty to eat, and then eat six of them in the car on the way home.

Toronto has an excellent bakery scene even if the bagel scene still sucks enough to make a trip to Montreal worth it. I don't typically look to the 905, or anyone who lives in that area code, for culinary recommendations, but The Banker's foodie colleague, Blake, has been raving about Monastery, and my sugar-seeking logic points out that *Blake* rhymes with *cake* and we had to pass through Oakville on our way back from visiting family in Hamilton anyway.

We pulled into the parking lot of a strip mall and found what appeared to be more of a medium-sized grocery than anywhere you'd expect to find Juliette Binoche. I wasn't getting monastery or bakery vibes, and it occurred to me that *Blake* also rhymes with *flake*. And *fake*. It's possible we'd been had.

"Are you sure this is the right place? It looks like where you buy communion wafers in bulk." I braced for disappointment when the automatic doors slid open and we were hit in the face with a blast of air conditioning instead of the smell of just-baked chocolate chip cookies. There was no antique bell announcing our arrival, just the beep of the checkout scanner and the crash of shopping carts slamming into the corral. But I tried to keep an open mind, because I really needed a snack.

Monastery turned out to be more of a gourmet grocer than the set of a rom-com. It's the kind of place you go to pimp out your charcuterie board with European specialty items like cornichons and soppressata. It's staffed with people who understand cheese. If you're looking for chips, they will be Parmesan or truffle flavoured, definitely cooked in a kettle. I could get excited about this.

"What do you think? Should we do a pass?" The Banker asked. I saw him notice the sample stations, free samples being a strong indicator that he would want to do at least two passes.

"Let's get a cart," I said, nodding. I had no intention of filling it, but grocery carts and baby strollers double as discreet entry-level mobility aids—a substitute for a walker, which I am not yet ready for (mentally, at least). "Maybe they'll have *turrón*," I said, knowing no one ever has the almond confection I fell in love with in Madrid. (Do not come at me with marzipan. It is not the same thing.)

I threw my cane in the cart and followed The Banker toward the first sample station.

"Would you like to try some olive oil?" an older man (older than me anyway) asked. "It's from Turkey. From my best friend, Omer's, grove."

"Cool," I said. "We have so much olive oil at home, though." It wasn't a lie; we have more than we can store and I didn't want to give Sample Guy hope for a sale, especially when he had a best-friend backstory. The Banker, not so much. He helped himself to a second sample.

"You should try this, Sheppy. It's really good."

"It won the Sol d'Oro," Sample Guy added, like it should mean something to me.

"In Rome."

Oh, well then. "It's very lovely. Thank you!" I said, ready to move on. "We should get some tapenade," I whispered to The Banker as I started walking. Tapenade isn't olive oil but it's olive oil–adjacent. "But first let's find the pastries."

The pastry section confirmed that Monastery is Italian-owned. Towered high, overflowing with cream. There were a dozen variations of cannoli and everything was labelled with a fancy foreign word ending with a vowel and a reverence for authenticity. Everything except the sad-looking mille feuilles I spied in the back of the case. It was labelled "custard slice" and they may as well have called it "basic."

"Stay away from the macarons," I warned. "I don't think the baker is fond of the French." I was ready to check out the cheese, but suddenly I had to pee.

"Can you take the cart and see if they have any of that good Dijon? I'll meet you back at the cheese in a bit." I didn't ask him to handle the cheese. Cheese decisions are my domain.

The Banker passed me back my cane and I realized how much I'd been relying on the cart. By the time I made it back to the dairy counter, I'd needed to sit down, but there was no chair or bench (or Banker) in sight. I sat on the edge of the fridge and tried to make it look like I was casually considering camemberts and bries. When I looked around to see where the fuck my husband was, I made eye contact with Sample Guy, twenty feet away. He waved and I smiled, while feeling mad at myself for having broken the no-eye-contact-with-someone-who's-trying-to-sell-you-something rule.

When The Banker finally returned, I handed him a wedge of Bella-Vitano and decided to call it a day. "Can I have the keys?" I said. "I'm gonna wait in the car."

"Take the cart," he offered, scooping up the groceries before heading to the checkout. I grabbed the handle and felt instantly 30 percent better.

As I passed Sample Guy on my way out, he stopped me. If his plan had been to divide and conquer, he should have targeted The Banker, who spends less freely than I do but has a way harder time telling anyone no.

"Miss?" he said.

"Mm-hmm?"

"You have MS."

Just like that. It wasn't a question, just a statement. No warm-up or small talk. It was almost spooky. I wanted to be pissed at what was a pretty bold observation, but I was too curious. Was this guy some kind of upselling sideshow psychic? Like, *Step right up to the Sensational Sample Guy! His remarkable clairvoyance can guess your age or ailment with unparalleled accuracy! Omer's Terrific Turkish Olive Oil will restore you to perfect health!*

"How did you know?" I asked, without considering that sitting in cheese might have been the first clue.

"I have MS too. Thirty years."

"Oh," I said, but this takes-one-to-know-one answer wasn't enough to satisfy me. I realize that people see my cane and draw their own conclusions, but this one was incredibly specific.

"I've done okay," he continued. "It's been slow-moving." It seemed true enough. I don't know how long he'd been standing at Omer's olive oil station, but he was standing. (Meanwhile, my feelings about Omer had shifted. Seems like kind of a douchey bestie, making his friend work so hard without even providing a chair.)

"Any words of wisdom?" I asked, because I didn't know what else to say. I was still processing the fact that a total stranger could identify me so easily. I didn't feel naked, but I did feel exposed.

Sample Guy's eyes were kind but intense. He held my gaze and it was unnerving. "I wish the best for you," he said, and I could tell he meant it, though I wasn't convinced he expects it. "I wish the best for you" sounds heavy on the wishing.

I found The Banker in line at the checkout counter and added a bottle of the Nostradamus's truth-telling oil to the belt, because I'm not taking any chances. Then I made my way to the car. From the passenger seat, I watched Sample Guy exit the store. He was now using a cane and I clocked his gait: slow, his right foot kind of dragging. I guess that's how I look too. He struggled to pull a suitcase on wheels. *Shoulda used a cart.*

I long ago accepted that I have a chronic illness—after all, I've had MS for more than fifteen years. Having an incurable disease versus having a disability might sound like semantics, but to me, the distinction is huge. Maybe it's hard to believe (unless you, too, have MS), but I've been rejecting the disabled label without ever actually considering it (despite living with some pretty disabling symptoms).

With the line between being sick and being disabled starting to blur, my identity starts to feel less up to me to decide. MS is no longer something I have (a disease), but something I am. I'm not just sick anymore, I'm sick and disabled.

31 / Say Something

DR. POKER FACE still takes my calls, but it's getting harder to make the trip to Hamilton to see him. It's time to find a neurologist in Toronto.

Dr. Roy-Hewitson floats into the exam room at St. Michael's Hospital—one of the world's biggest and most important MS clinics, and introduces herself as Chantal. I try to keep the bewilderment from registering on my face. I've spent fifteen years in Club MS and I don't have the nerve to call my new neurologist by anything other than her status-wielding professional designation. A warm and compassionate, young and energetic doctor who, for some reason, seems to think we're equals? The dynamic is so unfamiliar that it's unnerving, and when she tells me that I most certainly have secondary progressive MS (SPMS) and that it's time for me to get a walker—maybe even a scooter—I don't freak out. At least not immediately.

It's not shocking that I've left the relapsing remitting phase of MS, and now have so-called SPMS. I no longer respond to steroids and my symptoms seem to insidiously get worse without ever bouncing back. It is, however, a drag to hear it made official, especially when the designation significantly limits the treatment options that are available to me.

I dismiss the recommendation of a scooter outright, but I know "Chantal" is right about the walker. I take the note in my Frankensteinian stride. The thickening layer of handprints streaked across the walls of my apartment prove I'm no longer getting by with just a cane. A walker is a practical and prudent solution that will preserve some of my precious energy and keep me safe from unnecessary falls.

That evening, on one of the first warm Friday evenings in late spring, TB and I are having charcuterie and sangria on the balcony. I'm casually delivering the headlines from my day when suddenly all of my well-adjusted adjusting disappears. The sudden change in my perspective feels so unexpected that I know it must be poisonous. But I can't stop myself from picking it up and taking a big sip of hysteria, just like with the boozy juice sitting in front of me.

I'd left my new doctor's office feeling calm and mature for how I was processing the whole "progressive disability" thing. But now, regurgitating the intel, saying the words out loud to my husband, the words that communicate my need of a walker—a fucking *walker*—it all makes me feel like I'm having an out-of-body experience. I briefly lose my mind.

Living in slow-motion terror isn't easy. My panic feels like it's about the walker, but the walker is just the thing I can point to—the symbol, the bookmark of where I am in the story.

TB tries to calm me down, but I'm having none of it. He counters each of my anxieties with hopeful reassurances and hunks of baguette smeared with brie. He tells me for the millionth time that we are in this together and that his life is a billion times better with any version of me in it, while urging me to try the pâté. He pours more sangria, and that helps, but I can be very convincing, and finally I manage to make both of us cry.

I should be better at getting worse by now—after all, it's been fifteen years—but it's not like MS is a singular event. Knowing that my MS is now full-throttle secondary progressive is like being diagnosed all over again. I've only just come to terms with using a cane (that was supposed to be temporary, and technically, I guess it was), and now I have to get used to a walker? The stages of grief are useless when there's barely time to process one loss before another is piled on top.

The transition from walking to limping to using a cane and then a walker (and beyond), means ascending to a new level of disability each and every time. These are heartbreaking milestones that should come with presents or cake. But instead of pomp, there's only circumstance at disability graduations. A bump in my EDSS is the closest I'll get to any kind of diploma. There's not even a lousy postgrad keg party, because my friends and I are in our thirties. Nobody wants to stay up all night celebrating (or even acknowledging) anything so grim. Although drinking until I barf sounds pretty tempting right now.

I don't barf, but I do feel a bit better after half a pitcher of sangria and crying my eyes out, or at least I feel better for a while. When dealing with this kind of anguish, the first meltdown is rarely sufficient.

A few days later, my second wig-out in ten days leaves me feeling calmer again, but I'm still one meltdown away from turning the corner. The one where I ugly cry and insist I'm not strong enough. The one where TB tells me "it will get better" and I slam my fists and cry "it's never getting better" over and over until he seems to at least consider that I'm right, even if he doesn't accept it. Because the very worst part is never what's happening, but whatever it is that happens next.

I'm not sleeping, and I feel like a mess, but beyond The Banker, I don't know how to ask for help. I've been handling MS for so long that everyone assumes I have my shit together, that I know how to do this, but I'm not okay—because none of this is okay.

I spend weeks mired in anxiety and grief before I finally pour my heart out on the blog: it's a literal cry for help. I hear from other Trippers, but otherwise I'm screaming into the void. More than one person close to me tells me they saw my post but were too afraid to read it. I want to scream, *YOU NEED TO HEAR ME*, but my pain is too big, too complicated, too permanent for civilians. I'd forgotten that my job is to make MS as normal as possible, to make MS comfortable for everyone else. Those are the rules. I don't bother mentioning that this particular blog post starts rough but has a tidy feel-good ending—it's even foreshadowed in the post's title—because I know that if I'm too hard to be around, I will scare everyone away.

My loved ones aren't total assholes. From breakups to barren wombs to bankruptcy, everyone has multitudes of their own suffering, and everyone's living in some version of their own personal hell. My friends aren't therapists, they aren't anxiety meds, they're barely blog readers, and they're certainly not mind readers. I can't expect them to solve this crisis for me.

It takes weeks for my walker to arrive. In the meantime, I learn that we call them rollators now. The rebrand is a surprising comfort. *Rollator* doesn't conjure the image of a cartoon grandmother hunched over a bulky device. *Rollator* reminds me of my 1990s Rollerblades. Meanwhile, the impossibly slow health-care system causing the delay in delivering my new set of wheels gives me ample time to process this staggering new life change.

When my rollator finally arrives, I look at it and cry one more time at this ugly black machine that will be attached to every outfit in my foreseeable future. My D cups used to be the first thing to enter a room before me; now it's this clunky motherfucker, half my height and twice my width. Someone suggests I drape it in Christmas lights, like I'm seven, and also somehow an electrical outlet.

I do what I can to make the device less loathsome, to make it feel more like me. I remove anything that feels unnecessary and even some things I might need, like the outfit-blocking backrest, which is the first thing to go. It's wide and plastic and has the manufacturer's name branded on it in big white letters, like it was made by Prada or Marc Jacobs. The basket is enormous enough that it could hold several bottles of wine, but securing the family wine isn't my job so the basket gets tossed too. Next I cover the orange metal knobs on the handles with thirty-five dollars' worth of Dior nail polish in gunmetal grey. There's not much I can do about the orange plastic handle in the middle of the seat, but I tie a scarf around it until I can think of something better.

To be honest, I'm not that crafty, and I have no business being anywhere near Pinterest. I'm not much of a DIYer and it's entirely possible that I've transformed the rollator from something that looks new but ugly into something that still looks ugly and has also been stripped for parts. Whether or not my modifications are improvements is debatable, but what's certain is the middle finger I'm giving to the situation. My make-under is my way of saying, *I know I have to do this, but I sure as shit don't like it.*

A month later, I've calmed down substantially and am ready to see my family at my brother James's wedding. I'm nervous for a crowd of relatives and strangers to see me using a rollator. I dress as cheerfully as possible—this is not my day. My tea-length dress has spaghetti straps, a deep V-neck and layers of pale pastel stripes tied at the waist with a pink satin belt that matches my manicure. It's a feminine and confident look, but I still feel like I have to explain myself. "Remember me? Ardra? I guess you can see that I use a walker now, but actually we're calling them rollators. It's no big deal, so you don't have to be sad or whatever. Wasn't that a great dinner?"

I want to crawl into a hole, but there's an open bar, so I don't leave. Plus, it really is a beautiful day and a chance to celebrate my baby brother having found The One. His bride, Jenny, is funny and cool and pretty. She's sporty and adventuresome, but normal? Like, I'm kinda shocked that James found someone who can tolerate snakes living in the house. Then again, maybe she doesn't know. (As a kid, my reptile- and amphibian-loving brother was regularly caught with frogs and other creatures in his bedroom. In high school, he briefly housed a family of turtles in his locker.) I probably should have warned Jenny, but I already missed the whole speak-now-or-forever-hold-your-peace part. *Good luck, girl.*

By the time my sister, Corinne, and I have polished off a bottle of sparkling wine together, I feel emboldened to confess to how hurt I'd been that nobody had checked in with me after my gut-wrenching blog post.

"I think about you all the time, but I don't always know what to say," she says, truly and sincerely sorry.

"You don't have to fix it. I just need to hear 'Hey, I'm thinking of you, I know this is hard, I love you.'"

"You always do that for me," she says. "You deserve the same. I know this is hard. I do love you." I feel relieved and supported and grateful for this simple, alcohol-fortified exchange. Maybe I don't have to have my shit together all the time, I just need to be able to ask for what I need when I need it. I just wish that I didn't have to.

32 / What Now?

FOLLOWING MY TWO-YEAR TREATMENT with alemtuzumab, a.k.a. HSCT Lite, I get an email from the drug company's patient support program, soliciting feedback. They want to know how alemtuzumab, my fifth DMT—after four failed licensed therapies and two medical interventions in Poland—has made a difference in my life. They're offering me a twenty-five-dollar gift card for my trouble.

I know what kind of feedback the pharmaceutical company is hoping for. They want to hear that, thanks to their kick-ass drug, I went from being ruled by disease to routinely forgetting I even have MS. Instead of lying around watching *Gilmore Girls*, I'm hiking the Himalayas and crossing shit off my bucket list. I ditched my aquafit friends because those blue-haired geriatrics were holding me back. Now I teach dolphins to swim.

Never mind that I can't find the Himalayas on a map, I would never ditch Shirley, and dolphins are notorious jerks. I do the survey because I want that twenty-five bucks, but I suspect the drug company will be disappointed in my answers.

The question is, *How has alemtuzumab made a difference in your life?* And it's true, there have been some changes. My most obvious metamorphosis is that I have blonde hair now. Technically the drug didn't cause my de-pigmentation, but it is the first thing that anyone who hasn't seen me in a while notices. It's possible that "OMG you're a blonde now!" is more socially acceptable than "OMG you're using a walker!" but I like to think the walker isn't that noticeable.

Although the hope was that the drug would slow down my MS, maybe even encourage some small improvements, I walked into treatment using a cane only occasionally. Now I'm using a rollator on the regular. My EDSS jumped one whole point and I can no longer jump at all.

Meanwhile, my immune system has been reconstituted. My lymphocytes were murdered, and I guess they told their friends, because it's taking a long time for new ones to come back. Without sufficient white blood cells, my defences are down and I almost always have a UTI. If you sneeze within earshot, we will not be friends anymore.

Accepting the possibility of acquiring secondary autoimmune conditions due to treatment with certain medications is one of the deals with the devil that patients strike when they decide the risks of untreated MS are scarier than the risk of developing Graves' disease, opportunistic infections or some other mystery disorder. It's the reason why I'm required to have blood tests and urinalysis every month for the next four years. Post-alemtuzumab secondary autoimmunity is also the likely reason I developed a mast cell condition that has sent me to the ER multiple times covered in hives and in a state of anaphylaxis.

I don't regret my decision to have this treatment, though it was not my first choice. Many people have been treated with alemtuzumab and have had fantastic results. It's an amazing drug; it just wasn't amazing for me.

I show up for my final appointment with Dr. Muppet, wearing my best blazer in an attempt to be taken seriously.

"So, what now?" I ask, already knowing that he isn't willing to move forward with our original plan B, the one where he said that if I failed this drug, he'd give me HSCT. Dr. Muppet had been dismissive of my worsening symptoms at all of my follow-up appointments, so I'm not holding my breath.

"If HSCT Lite didn't work, HSCT won't work either" is Dr. Muppet's unfeeling reply. I don't disbelieve it. HSCT Lite might have kept me from having attacks but it also feels like it somehow accelerated my decline.

Perhaps the good news is not what's different after alemtuzumab, but what's the same. My MRIs are stable; there's no new inflammation. I haven't had new attacks (yet). In 2015, Dr. Muppet doesn't talk to me about why some patients experience disease progression in the absence of relapses. The concept of so-called smouldering MS isn't a term I will hear for a few more years, once the medical community starts to better understand the disease. In the meantime, what he does say feels cruel and unnecessary.

"If you'd come to me ten years ago, I'd have given you HSCT."

Thinking about what could have been stings even if it doesn't feel like he's telling the truth. Didn't he tell me at my first appointment—*two years ago*—that the patients he treats with HSCT show up with a higher EDSS than the one I'd had when he first assessed me? The number that's much closer to my EDSS now?

With no more drugs for me to try and nothing left to do but wait for something better, something that might never come, I feel sidelined, abandoned, hopeless. I leave Ottawa in despair. Even though nobody will look me in the eye and say it out loud, it feels like it's only a matter of time before I can't use my legs at all, and why the fuck isn't everyone (or anyone) freaking out about it?

33 / I See You Looking

AFTER GRADUATING HIGH SCHOOL back in the 1990s, I was heartbroken that a lack of francs meant I had to abandon my post-secondary plan A to study voice in Paris. I'd been accepted at the Sorbonne, but I didn't have the financing to live abroad, and so I enrolled at Montreal's McGill University instead.

Of course, Montreal didn't deserve my disappointment. Canada's coolest city, Montreal can only be considered a consolation prize in comparison to Paris. It helped that my then-boyfriend, The Very Tall One, was going to McGill as well. With its cobblestones and distinctive francophone culture, if I squinted (and drank enough red wine), I could convince myself that Montreal was in Europe anyway.

At nineteen, I dreamt of becoming an opera singer and of living a bourgeois lifestyle. I wanted to travel the world, speak six languages, drink champagne with artsy original thinkers. Montreal felt like a place where I could cultivate who I thought I was and wanted to be: worldly, cultured, classy, cool.

I arrived at McGill anxious to start dressing in black and acting like *une vraie Montréalaise,* except for taking up smoking (I was a singer, after all). I couldn't wait to buy a Metro pass, the flimsy plastic passport to my future that would turn me into a card-carrying urbanite. To this day, the stale urine-scented air of the underground, coupled with the screech of trains, and the occasional rat sighting, is my Proustian madeleine—a sensory experience I long for. That carcinogenic metallic musk means I'm in New York, London or Paris—someplace exciting, at a time, at least, when I could still handle a little pushing and shoving, and a few flights of stairs.

Unfortunately, a chic new wardrobe was not in my student-loan budget. I mostly lived in the same pair of green track pants—the paint-splattered ones with the tiny hole in the knee—and three layers of sweaters, because my slumlord refused to adequately heat my apartment.

Instead of champagne, I was drinking tap water and off-brand Coke, hoping I wouldn't get food poisoning from the 49 Cent Slice. I realized I would have to pay my dues as a *bohème* before I could graduate to the bourgeoisie. While I waited to be rich and famous, I decided to focus on growing my circle of artsy original friends.

An unlikely first contender was the girl renting a room in the same apartment as me. My new roommate was a waif-like blue-eyed natural blonde, with a carpet of leg hair to prove it. A physics brainiac, Blue Eyes had a sweet girlish voice and a humility that made her easy to underestimate. I immediately wanted to give her a makeover, but Blue Eyes had no interest in conforming. Her *au naturel* look was a long-term fuck you to some kid in grade school who'd told her she'd have great legs if only she would shave them. She told that kid that, thanks to him, she wouldn't shave her legs for the rest of her goddamn life. But it was this chick's veganism that made her truly exotic to me.

Obviously I knew about vegetarians. I even knew one personally. But I had never heard of anyone who didn't eat cheese; and fine, judge me, but again, this was the nineties. There were no vegans on TV. I'd only just discovered avocados, and kale had yet to be invented.

There weren't any gay people on TV either, though I also knew they existed. As a future diva, I aspired to be a gay icon someday. But imagining myself as the Madonna of opera didn't stop me from doing a dramatic double take the first time I saw two guys holding hands on the Metro. Awestruck, I actually gawked. I'd never seen gay PDA and I felt like I'd seen a unicorn. Well, two unicorns.

As a nineties teen, my interpretation of grunge meant pairing my Catholic school uniform with heavy eyeliner and my precious eight-hole Docs. I knew every *Downward Spiral* lyric by heart, but I had zero chill about the goth in the back of Anthropology 101 who wore a Nine Inch Nails T-shirt and a six-inch nail through his eyebrow. This was not the kind of preppy post-secondary student the J.Crew catalogue had prepared me for. I don't know what the hell Margaret Mead ever did because I couldn't take my eyes off of Trent Reznor long enough to listen to any of the lectures.

The encounter that undid me, though, was with my new friend Leigh. He was an engineering student, a pot-smoking, recreational race-car driver from small-town Nova Scotia. Tall (we grow them big in Canada), with a mess of floppy hair, Leigh wasn't a contender for my salon of artsy original thinkers. Leigh was an ordinary guy. He was friends with The Very Tall One, which meant we were only close-adjacent. Close enough anyhow that when I had my wisdom teeth removed and wondered if vodka would make my prescription pain meds work better, Leigh delivered an impassioned speech about the risks of liver failure; and when his parents came to town, I was included in his my-parents-want-to-meet-my-friends brunch.

I was already sitting at our favourite greasy diner, La Belle Province, with The Very Tall One and Mike, when Leigh arrived. Leigh wasn't hard to spot as he made his way toward us, clearing space for a man half his size who was hunched over on two forearm crutches. Leigh: the kind of guy who prevents you from poisoning yourself and helps the disabled fight their way through hordes of hungover teens.

"Hey, guys," said Leigh as he arrived at the booth with the hobbling man. "These are my parents." I hadn't yet noticed the woman who was now taking the crutches from her husband as he settled into the end of the booth. I was stunned. *Why didn't Leigh tell us his dad had had polio? Why didn't he warn us?*

My friends and I ordered pancakes and crappy coffee. We politely asked Leigh's parents about their trip to Montreal. Like most of our own dads, Leigh's dad was proud of his kid, prone to bad jokes and told mildly embarrassing stories about what his son was like as a child. It was just another Sunday at the diner, but having a meal with someone disabled made a lasting impression on me. I don't know what I expected, but what I experienced can only be described as . . . totally normal.

Leigh never spoke to me about his father's disability, which had the effect of rendering the intel irrelevant. By saying nothing, the message was clear that his father's health wasn't an issue, and furthermore, none of my business.

For all my self-perceived worldliness, Montreal had exposed me as a slack-jawed country bumpkin. As ignorant as every other kid who'd just been released from their suburban childhood prisons. Without saying anything, Leigh had taught me a valuable lesson. Not that I think Leigh was trying to teach me anything. Leigh was just living his life.

33

I can't pretend that Montreal cured me of my weirdness. I'm sure there have been plenty of times over the years when I've been inadvertently guilty of othering someone who looks different from me. I'll never know if Trent Reznor, Leigh's dad or the subway unicorns ever noticed my double takes. Even if they'd all been oblivious (and I doubt I was that subtle), each would have encountered rubberneckers like me before. I know, because now I'm someone who gets gawked at too.

Intent matters, and curiosity isn't the same as contempt, but I have yet to cultivate the kind of chill that doesn't leave me rattled when I see someone looking.

34 / What's Wrong With *Me*? What's Wrong With *You*?

IMAGINE THE HARDEST THING you've ever gone through. Now imagine that people who don't even know your name want you to tell them what that is.

I've been fielding questions about my body ever since I started using a cane, and it's only ramped up since I began using a rollator. *What's wrong with your leg? Why are you walking like that? What happened to you?* I get it. People aren't used to seeing people like me—young but using the tools of the old—and some of these people want answers.

I don't believe that everyone who asks about my disability is a nosy jerk, but *What's wrong with you?* is not an acceptable icebreaker.

Recently I was trapped in an elevator with an elderly man who gestured to my rollator and said, "I'm glad I don't need one of those." Way to go, old guy! Finding gratitude in your day! Though his appreciation did not make me feel better.

Once, when a curious stranger gave me the up-down before declaring, "You're too young to be using one of those," Fantasy Me said, *You're too old to be asking rude questions.* But Reality Me just didn't respond.

I don't even know how to feel about the time a guy pulled over to ask me where he could donate the wheelchair he was driving around with.

The uncomfortable behaviour of strangers isn't limited to invasive Qs and less-than-brilliant observations either. People regularly hurl themselves in front me as I get close to an elevator, swooping in to push the button like they're taking a bullet for me. One time, a guy in my building did this, then gave me three pats on the back.

I wish I could tell you that the last time someone tried to tie my shoelace was when I was four years old, but The Banker is not immune to prying eyes. Sometimes when we're out he'll do shit for me that he would never do at home because he knows people are watching and he doesn't want to be judged as the guy who lets a disabled woman fend for herself.

All of this peacockery isn't so much to help me as it is to show me that the peacocks care, that they want to help, that they're one of the good guys. And how can I be mad at that? We need people who care.

These conspicuous but basically useless actions are collectively known as virtue signalling. Never mind that virtue signalling often leaves targets feeling more othered than included. We all do it.

Okay, maybe not everyone. If you're one of those man-spreaders on the subway who pretends not to notice that someone needs your seat, this message isn't for you. Go back to your cave.

I want people to know I'm an ally—that I support diversity, religious freedom and LGBTQIA+ communities, and sometimes I overdo it. Like the time my white ass considered sporting a head scarf to "support" my hijab-wearing Muslim girlfriend who was being continually harassed on the subway. Fortunately, I didn't actually do this, but I did think about it out loud. (I'm so sorry, Sadaf!) It's just like that misguided COVID celebrity singalong: The last thing I want is to inadvertently condescend to anyone who doesn't enjoy the privileges I do. Like Will Ferrell's confusing performance of "Imagine," my heart was in the right place.

But good intentions don't mean micro-aggressions are harmless. If you get only one mosquito bite a year, you might be tempted to let it slide. If you are swarmed by mosquitoes every time you leave the house, you might consider bathing in DEET and wrapping yourself in protective netting.

Although virtue signalling feeds our own egos and identities, telling people we're on their side doesn't actually do anything to effect change (#IAmCharlie but I can't remember why). But just because you're virtue signalling doesn't mean you don't care. In fact, you probably do care (terrorism = bad, satire = good).

I don't speak for everyone with a disability, or for everyone with MS, for that matter. Lots of people believe that kindness shouldn't be questioned. I don't want to succumb to the stereotype of Bitter Disabled Person, but I don't want to feel like the Grateful Inspiration stereotype either. I resent the notion that I have to be performatively indebted and appreciative for whatever's thrown at me, whether I need it or not.

The good news is that most of us have got each other's backs. We're getting better at this whole being human thing. What I want all the concerned randos I encounter to know is that it's not sympathy I'm after. It's not pats on the back or applause. We don't see enough real diversity in media, especially when it comes to sickness, so when we see it IRL, we draw from what we've learned from *Forrest Gump* or *Frankenstein* and the effed-up biases we don't even know we have. The path to being a true ally involves getting to know someone who's different—on social media, in real life and through quality storytelling.

If you still want to express your concern for me, then advocate for accessible transit, hire someone with a disability, be fucking outraged that most bars and restaurants in Toronto, Montreal, New York, London and Paris are still not accessible. Demand better content and more diverse stories from the culture-makers—the kinds of stories that might give us all a healthier, less stereotypical perspective on people who are different from us.

And if all that's too much, then just be normal. We all deserve to be here.

35 / How I Roll

"IS THIS HAT TOO MUCH OR NOT ENOUGH?" I ask my friend Lisa about the torso-sized top hat that's perched on my head. It's a good thing I have my rollator for balance or I might tip over.

"Of course it's too much! It's perfect!" she yells so that she can be heard over the crowd and the music. "Look at these freaks!" she says, waving her arms at the nineteen hundred or so Gothic pirates dressed almost exclusively in black, their outfits accessorized with lace, round glasses, corsets and aviation goggles. We're not at a rave, we're at a gala fundraiser where the dress code is steampunk. The Art Gallery of Ontario (AGO) has been transformed from a quiet and airy space into something dark and club-like. It's the kind of event designed to make you feel like an insider, though it seems to be populated with outsiders.

Before we reach the bar, two strangers stop to compliment me on the vintage hat I've borrowed from my mom's extensive millinery collection. On the heels of my brother's wedding, this gala is my second large-scale function with my rollator as my date, and a focus-stealing hat provides an extra bit of armour.

Putting a hat on a hat may not be an effective way to minimize stares, but dressing less like myself and more like I'm playing a character lets me indulge the warped belief that I'm not really a disabled woman who needs mobility aids to get around. It's not a tough sell to my psyche. I'm still struggling to reconcile that the way I look on the outside doesn't match how I feel on the inside. Catching my reflection, I still find myself doing double takes when I don't immediately recognize the mobility-aid version of myself.

The civil war between the body I *had* and the body I *have* has been playing out for months in a recurring dream. While I'm asleep, I walk for miles through the streets of Paris. Sometimes I'm even running, and it all feels so easy. I assume my subconscious is confused and frustrated, that my dreaming brain is trying to remind my body of how it's supposed to move. It places me in Paris to maximize the incentive.

This is the look-at-me/don't-look-at-me energy I'm rocking when some media type approaches and asks if he can take my picture. He tells me my hat caught his eye, and suddenly feeling cool again, I'm happy to oblige.

"Hold my drink," I tell Lisa, as I grab the cane that's attached to my rollator and shove the rollator out of the way. I touch up my lipstick and cautiously work my angles.

BEFORE I'M EVEN OUT OF BED the next morning, I do what any proper party girl does and sift through four hundred megabytes of selfies, deleting any that are blurry, where my hair looks less than perfect, where my resting bitch face is uncalled for. I know I'm a good person, because I delete the snaps where my friends look subpar too. Women supporting women.

Twenty-two photos get dragged to trash immediately because my lazy left eye makes me look drunk or sleepy. I was probably a bit of both, but I'm not interested in photorealism. I narrow my options to three or four, scrutinizing the subtle differences, then upload the winner to my social media so that I can share my glam and exciting life, all before brushing my teeth.

When I suddenly remember the professional-looking photographer who paparazzi'd me last night, I put off making coffee to see if I made the Toronto equivalent of *Page Six*. I scan *The Kit* and *BlogTO*, then check the AGO's Instagram, swiping through stories, scanning hashtags that might accompany a hat four times the size of my head. I find dozens of shots of happy revellers, but I can't find any of me. I keep coming up empty. *Dammit, why didn't I ask Slim Aarons who the eff he works for?* A true It Girl, of course, would be too cool to care.

Then it hits me. *Happy memory, happy memory, uh-oh memory.* You know the kind that presents itself once you've sobered up enough to creep your mental inventory of just what happened during a night of drinking? The process of scanning for shame—*Who did you drunk-text? Who did you wake up next to? Who did you offend?*

Under a disco ball and the influence of more than one cucumber martini, I had pretended not to know, or need, my rollator, for the sake of the photo. And sure, I didn't punch anyone, make out with a stranger or spill any embarrassing secrets, but I still had the crushing morning-after realization that I may have offended a mobility aid, *my* mobility aid; and maybe my rollator isn't sentient, but it is the thing that's attached to me, the thing I depend on to get around. In a fucked-up way, by dissing my rollator, I kind of dissed myself.

I've been shoving my rollator out of pictures since it arrived on my doorstep, and before that I was ditching my cane for pics that were private and never intended for a magazine or even a blog. In documenting my own life, I'm not trying to rewrite history. Selfies help us influence how we are perceived by others, but what about how we perceive ourselves? I kicked my rollator out of the frame out of fear of how strangers will judge me. I also happen to think I look better without my hands on a mobility aid. Like everyone else, I've been brainwashed into interpreting mobility aids as symbols of my brokenness.

Unless I want to continue feeling diminished by something I can kind of hide but cannot change, I need to decide that "disabled" is a look I can rock. It's hard to accept that disability can be normal and even beautiful, because we never see it represented that way. I had a chance to prove it last night and I totally fucking blew it.

I have such a chip on my shoulder about the stigma around mobility aids that it never occurred to me that the hat might not have been what was most interesting about me, or that my mobility aid may not have been what was most egregious. Maybe what caught Camera Guy's eye was the whole picture, the sum of my parts. Or maybe I was just another one of nineteen hundred people and I need to get over myself.

The best version of me doesn't hide my disability, but handles it with grace. Unfortunately, I'm still a work in progress. I can't promise I won't do it again.

36 / Can I Pray for You?

DESPITE WHAT MY SOCIAL MEDIA would have you believe, I'm normally dressed like Relic from *The Beachcombers*. If I'm not leaving the house or going anywhere near a camera, I'm rocking a look that suggests maybe I, too, live on a tugboat without access to a washing machine. My go-to uniform is old-ass track pants, two pairs of socks and the T-shirt I slept in. If it's colder than twenty-three degrees Celsius inside my apartment, I'll throw on fingerless gloves and a tattered knit cap to complete the look. I love fashion, but I spend most of my life at home with the dog, hoping nobody shows up unexpectedly.

Today, though, is an "outside world" day. My nails are done and someone else has washed and blow-dried my hair. I'm wearing heirloom pearls and garnet earrings, and I've tucked an embroidered hanky in my leather clutch instead of stuffing a wad of gently used Kleenex up my sleeve. My most important accessory is my brand-new ivory-coloured rollator—the bougiest mobility aid on the market. I look shiny, like I have all my shit together. I'm overdressed for Branch 58. And sure, even jeans with a belt would be overdressed for the east end Hamilton Legion, but it's the day of my grandfather's funeral and I'm not looking to fit in.

Anyway, I'll still be two degrees south of Human Peacock compared to my more-is-more mother, who never misses an opportunity to be the most extravagant person in the room. I fully expect Norma to show up to her father-in-law's funeral looking like a grieving Janet Jackson, shrouded in a black lace veil and a hat so enormous that, if tilted at the right angle, it would cause a local eclipse.

I can't speak for Norma, but the look I'm going for is Unapproachable Chic—a hug repellant for Uncle Inappropriate, who kisses everyone on the mouth, and a small-talk disincentive for anyone else who's not in my immediate inner circle. I've never been a fan of crowded spaces and super-spreader events, but I need an extra layer of armour to get through a day when I'm going to encounter a hundred people who've not yet seen me attached to a mobility aid, never mind that it's a fancy one. I'm not interested in fielding questions about my decline, or reassuring all these sad faces that I'm okay. I don't have the energy to repeatedly have the same conversation, and I'd rather tongue-kiss Uncle Inappropriate than listen to Uncle Ignorant tell me again how my bad attitude and love of sugar are the causes of my MS.

I leave Toronto in mint condition, feeling smug about choosing to chew my caffeine via a handful of chocolate-covered espresso beans rather than risk spilling coffee on my crisp white shirt. I nonetheless manage to snag my tights getting in the car. I may *look* like I have my shit together, but I'm still a clumsy hot mess at heart. It's fine. We have time. (We don't.) The Banker drops me off at the mall so I can grab a new pair of nylons while he goes to get gas.

"Get some cash for the after-party," I add. "You know it's not gonna be an open bar."

"Wake. You mean wake," he says. "It's not an after-party, God." But I'm already rollatoring toward the mall.

Fifteen minutes later, I'm sitting on my rollator, two pairs of new tights in hand, waiting for The Banker. It's windy and I don't wanna wreck my hair, so I'm perched just inside the door when a smiling woman approaches. She's young—probably in her twenties—a detail that feels meaningless at first.

"Excuse me. Can I ask you a question?"

"Of course," I reply with genuine warmth because I'm still naive and have jumped to the conclusion that she obviously wants to know about my new high-end rollator. I get asked about it a lot, and I imagine her proudly pulling up the device's website to tell one of her grandparents about the cool lady she saw with the sick device. I'm about to launch into the benefits of carbon fibre and hidden cables when she reaches toward me with both hands and asks, "Can I pray for you?"

Wait. What? I'd heard about these sneak-attack intercessions, but it's the first time I've experienced one in the wild. I try to process the thrill of witnessing what had, until this moment, felt like an urban legend, but my impulse to recoil is stronger than my curiosity. My body moves away from the woman, but there is nowhere to go. My rollator is parked against the wall and I am trapped.

"No, thanks. I'm okay," I reply with a furrowed brow and an expectation that my refusal will sufficiently motivate her to move on. The downtown mall is so popular with the disabled crowd that there are handmade signs posting speed limits for power chairs on every other corner. It shouldn't take her long to find someone else to save.

"God wants you to be better," she says with the kind of authority that suggests she has a direct line to Jesus. She's doubling down and I am not prepared for a standoff. Maybe if I was wearing my fingerless gloves like some shivering Dickensian orphan, I'd understand why she feels compelled to single me out as a tragic figure. I curse myself for having left my Prada sunglasses in the car.

Better from what? is what I *want* to say, to force her to articulate just what she thinks is wrong with me. I can't imagine my need for a mobility aid is any worse than whatever's going on in her life—in anyone's, for that matter. But you don't see me trolling the mall telling people that a Higher Power thinks they need fixing, if only they'd let me put in a good word with the Big Guy on their behalf.

"Really, I'm fine." My smile is tense, but it's still a smile. I stand up to make myself taller, so that she can't physically look down on me. My precious rollator is now between us in case she tries to put her hands on me again.

"Don't you want to be cured?" she asks, like God is some kind of wish-granting genie. Her tone has travelled from pity to hostility now that it's clear I'm not willing to be her good deed for the day. The prayer I actually need is some version of: *Dear Lord, grant me the strength not to feel reduced by this missionary's misguided pity. Fill her targeted ads with opportunities to volunteer, donate or advocate for the disabled people she cares so deeply about. Help me find the strength of character to overlook her lack of common sense. In the meantime, thank you for the limited upper-body strength that prevents me from punching her directly in the twat.*

If I had a do-over, I would have folded my hands, bowed my head and said my prayer out loud.

"I have to go. My husband is waiting," I lie. I'd rather hang out on the street and ruin my blowout than suffer this conversation one second longer. Pity is not the same as empathy. Virtue signalling is not the same as building a ramp.

Still rattled, I remind myself that this day isn't about me. (*Do I, though?*) I join my siblings at the Legion, where the walls are still stained nicotine yellow despite the years that have passed since indoor smoking was banned. There are platters of Wonder Bread sandwiches, rolled-up cold cuts and cans of Lakeport at the bar. It's a place from a different time, haunted by the ghosts of a former bustling social scene. To us, the venue is synonymous with the salty retired steelworker and World War II vet we called Grampa, even if we got to see the inside of the building only once a year.

For all we knew, Grampa lived at the Legion. In the summer, our father would disappear into the mysterious brick building to have a drink with the man he was more likely to call Lloyd than Dad, leaving my sister, brother and me in the blue Ford van that served as our babysitter. I'd entertain myself with a book while Cory and James fought over the Game Boy until the battery died. Eventually, Grampa would appear with bags of ketchup chips, candy, cans of Orange Crush and Nevada tickets: the cardboard rectangles that introduced us to the excitement of a little light gambling.

But the Legion's annual kids' Christmas parties were a peek behind the curtain, which dispelled any *Charlie and the Chocolate Factory* fantasies we might have had about where all that candy was coming from. It was just a generic hall, decorated with the same gaudy decorations every year: an artificial Christmas tree stationed strategically in front of the accordion wall that would be tucked to the side, making room for the Chicken Dance we would be forced to endure for the amusement of our elders.

Grampa acted like he ran the place, making the rounds and shaking hands with everyone, and as the Legion's president for so many years, I guess he kind of did. Always on the lookout for his next potential wife, he flirted with all the ladies. As the grandkids of the Grand Poobah, we got preferential treatment. He'd slip us extra chocolate coins and make sure we got the good ice cream cups with the tiny wooden spoons (strawberry or chocolate swirl) before they ran out and all that was left was vanilla.

The Chicken Dance was humiliating but, by all accounts, worth it for the red mesh stocking—one for each kid—that always held a box of Cracker Jacks, two clementines, and three walnuts in the toe. We loved those parties and looked forward to them every year.

We pour one out for Grampa, the man who's the reason why any of us are here. When a young cadet nobody's heard of takes to the podium to gush about what a great guy Lloyd Shephard was, it's a reminder that the old man had status here. I assume he did the best he could, but calling him "great" feels like a stretch. Grampa was a good-time guy, but he had his demons. He wasn't a great dad, and he was pretty shitty to my sister at one point. I don't know who was praying for Grampa, a dedicated drinker, gambler and womanizer, but his ninety-four years proved that hard living and a lack of virtue didn't seem to take any years off his life.

My dad's eulogy is more nuanced. He talks about the man who, every year, tirelessly sold poppies to raise money for mobility aids and assistive devices for veterans and their families; who, regardless of his health or the weather, marched in every Remembrance Day parade to honour his fallen comrades; and who would show up at Hamilton's City Hall to advocate for veterans and seniors. He talks about the man who always had a pocketful of handwritten jokes to pull out after dinner, his raspy voice forcing us to lean in closer for the punchline.

My dad's grace reminds me that you can be kinda shitty and still be kinda great.

Two Lakeports in, Cousin Melodrama gets up to give a toast, and my sister and I exchange a "this should be good" look. My mom snorts, but her fucking veil gives her identity plausible deniability. We're pretty sure we're about to hear a poem, or an a cappella version of some contextually inappropriate song, like "I Will Always Love You" or "I Touch Myself." Awkward family moments are the best thing about weddings and funerals and I feel grateful to have siblings to share inside jokes with.

Grampa laughed easily, but he had a hard time saying "I love you." I don't profess to have known my grandfather well. I certainly didn't know him as an alcoholic absent father. I do know that, in a fucked-up way, Grampa is the reason why my own father never misses an opportunity to tell me he loves me and is proud of me.

The Grampa I knew would well up with tears whenever he heard me sing. I'm told that the first time he laid eyes on me as a baby, he said, "Even her ears are perfect." And when he saw me start to use a walker in my thirties, it brought him to tears again.

When I'd hear how he felt about my "goddamn disease," I'd shake my head in wonder. I don't expect to live anywhere near ninety-four years, but I have so many blessings—more blessings than the guy who grew up in poverty as one of thirteen mouths to feed, and who lied about his age as a teen to fight in a war. How can someone whose own life was so hard be brought to tears over my own?

Grampa dished out candy like a human vending machine for decades, which meant Grampa's excessive sentimentality was something I could let slide. And anyway, Grampa's tears were never performative or patronizing. I never had to say, *I'm okay, nothing to cry about over here*, because I heard about those tears only from others. I never saw them myself.

I don't want anyone to look at me and be sad. Pity, like the kind I got at the mall, doesn't make me feel loved and cared for, only misunderstood and othered. But I know Grampa's tears were not about pity. Whether I was sick or singing, when he struggled to find the right words, the old man's eyes, brimming with salt water, were his way of saying "I love you."

37 / Good Man

"SORRY, TRACE, I CAN'T TAKE ONE MORE BITE." I'm full of steak *frites* and *fromage*, and I had my heart set on the crème brûlée but my tummy just can't take it.

"Just the invoice, then," Tracy tells the waitress. Tracy means "the cheque," but she runs her own business now and "invoice" is the language of her people.

"One bill?" the waitress asks, gesturing to Tracy and her husband, Chris.

"Yes, please."

"And separate bills for you?" It's not the first time The Banker and I have been asked if we wanted individual bills. This server assumes Tracy and Chris are clearly a couple, but that The Banker and I are not.

"No, we're together," I say. She seems confused and requests confirmation.

"So, two bills? One for these two, and one for each of you?" she asks, eyebrows raised, like it's complicated.

When she leaves I want to say, *Can you believe that just happened?* But it's clear that no one has picked up on what I'm convinced is the waitress's assumption that my disability makes me an unlovable gargoyle, and that The Banker must be a distant cousin or a work colleague or someone equally uncommitted to sharing the cost of our dinner.

I decide not to let the interaction ruin my champagne buzz. We double-kiss Tracy and Chris as they get up to leave, and I brace myself for what comes next: my dramatic exit.

My disability enters every room before I do, announcing itself like it's the only thing worth knowing about me. The crowded bistro is too cramped to accommodate a rollator, so I use a cane and The Banker's arm to force my way through a maze of tables and busy waiters while muttering, "Excuse me" and "I'm sorry"—for being in the way, for being inconvenient, for things that aren't my fault. I'm not in the habit of mean-girling myself, and I'm grateful to be walking at all, but I know my walking isn't cute. It's bent and twisted, unsteady and insecure. Wherever I go, my stride draws stares of fascination and concern, stares that I swear I can physically feel. I know how uncomfortable it makes people to watch me walk, and yet nobody seems to look away.

I try telling myself I'm not making a scene, that it's self-indulgent to think everyone in the room is absorbed in my struggle to get to the door, when a diner two tables away, in a tone of admiration that's bordering on reverence, calls out to The Banker—who's right behind me, not doing anything special—"You're a good man."

At least this guy realizes TB and I are a couple, even if he doesn't seem to appreciate that I have ears and a brain—that I can hear him. I'm feeling even more wounded now. The Banker *is* a good man, maybe even the best man. But all this dude knows is that a guy who looks like he almost certainly works at a bank is out with a moderately disabled woman. He's so impressed by our togetherness that he feels compelled to publicly compliment it, the implication being that there is something extraordinary about a man like The Banker being with someone like me: the lucky girl this virtuous guy took pity on.

I know it shouldn't matter what other people think. I even know I'm overreacting. Maybe I'm sensitive to these micro-aggressions because they reinforce my nagging fear that I am, in fact, a burden. MS is a raw deal, not just for me but for TB too.

I save my thoughts for Darcy. We're due for a phone call anyway. "What an ass," she says, first about the waiter and then again, but louder, about the diner. She doesn't try to convince me of the goodness of humanity or that I'm imagining micro-aggressions, or that I should just shake it off. She lets me vent and now I can move on.

"I saw your Facebook update. Is that the first time you've posted a picture in your chair?" I ask, only sort of changing the subject. I've seen Darcy in her wheelchair in real life, but the social-media reveal was startling. It was bold. I'm freaking out about being seen with a cane, and I'm hiding my mobility aids in photos; meanwhile, Darcy's wheelchair is on display for every ex-lover, former high-school rival, friend of her mother or rando she ever Facebook-friended to gawk at.

"It's hard for Gracie."

"She's how old now?"

"Ten, going on twenty-five."

"She's a good kid. She'll come around. How's the dating scene?"

"It's a shit show. Ard, you are so lucky to have dodged online dating."

"So I've heard."

"I started posting the chair in my profile so that there wouldn't be any surprises. But I'm not just weeding out creepers and dick pics. I have to screen for disability 'devotees'—fetishists with a disability Fuck-It List."

"Seriously?"

"It's a thing."

"Barf. I don't know how you stand it."

"I don't. I'm sitting. Wine helps."

"What's the hardest part?"

"The guys who aren't sure if I can have sex because of the wheelchair, but they're afraid to ask. I feel like I need to open every conversation with: *Hi, I'm Darcy. Everything works.* They're so afraid to say the wrong thing and offend me, which ends up offending me more. Like, just ask what you wanna ask."

"Okay, cringe."

"Right? The worst, though, is if they use the word *cripple*."

"I can't believe anyone still thinks you can say 'cripple.'"

"Yeah, that's a hard pass."

"Totally *lame*," I add, and Darcy laughs. "What about the ones who can't roll with MS? That has to burn."

"The first time someone told me MS was a deal-breaker I was shocked. I didn't think anyone would actually say it to me. But, of course, he had every right to."

"After everything you went through with your marriage, you still believe in 'happily ever after'?"

"Absolutely. Maybe not 'in sickness and in health,' but we were so young. I don't blame him. Not anymore."

When Darcy's marriage became a casualty of her MS, it didn't surprise me: her high-school sweetheart couldn't handle the heat as her symptoms started to take over. What struck me was that Darcy was the one to leave. In her thirties, she decided she'd rather be a single mother, alone, than stick it out in a subpar marriage. By that point she was already a full-time wheelchair user with a reduced capacity to work. I feel like I'm supposed to glaze over the part where *she* left *him*. But it made her a fucking rock star to me.

"Damn, Darcy. When did you get so wise? When we got married, 'in sickness and in health' was not included in the first draft of the vows the officiant gave us and I made him put it back in."

"Oh my god, what were we thinking?" Darcy says.

"I wasn't trying to trap anyone! I think I just wanted him to publicly decree that I was worth the risk. That he knew what he was getting into."

"As if that's possible." I can practically hear her rolling her eyes.

"Yeah, vows are stupid. I believe in marriage, but I don't want a hostage situation—I want us both to stay because we want to, not because we have to."

"None of this is fun. It's work," she says. "I know I might have to go on a lot of bad dates—terrible dates—before I find him. But I know he's out there and that he's looking for me too," she adds, with the commitment of Meg Ryan circa 1995.

"I might know someone," I say. My friend Ryan is one of the few (only?) single guys I know who's looking for an actual relationship.

"What's he like?"

"Educated, curious, generous." I leave out the dad jokes and the incessant blinking. "He's blond," I add, gagging on the word. There's something about an adult man with natural blond hair that's disturbing to me.

"Would you date him?" she asks.

The question catches me off guard. I could probably get over the blinking, and most guys aren't as funny as they think they are. Darcy isn't put off by towheads, but her question makes me blush. "He's not my type" is a cliché that covers the intangible, hard-to-articulate ways in which Ryan would never make it past the friend zone with me. I suspect the same would be true for Darcy. She knows her MS narrows her dating options, but she doesn't think she has to settle for anything less than she's ever expected—someone who's smart, cool and fun. Someone with the charisma of Tom Hanks, and who's as hot as she is.

"No. You're right," I say. "Let's find you a smoke show." But Darcy doesn't need any help from me. Darcy doesn't need help from anyone.

38 / *xoJane*

TRIPPING ON AIR is becoming popular in the online MS community. People from around the world are leaving comments, sending me messages, telling me they feel seen. The response is thrilling, but when I tell my sister, Corinne, that I feel like an imposter calling myself a writer, she says, "Well, yeah, you're not a writer, you're a blogger." *Touché.*

Whatever this is—writing, blogging, oversharing on the internet—I'm discovering that I like putting words on the page. I'm not sure why this is news to me when I've kept a diary my whole life. Working on *Tripping on Air* is so fulfilling that I'm hardly thinking about the fact that I'm not singing. Finding *le mot juste* is as satisfying as nailing a high C (not to mention a lot more attainable these days). Even the moment I hit "publish" sometimes feels like a bit of a Stage Door Day.

Blogging is rewarding, but maybe my sister is picking up on something, because I don't want to be just a blogger. I want to see what else my voice can do. Maybe it's "real" writing, maybe it's something else.

I start pitching to various online publications. I pen some chronic-illness content for *The Mighty*. It doesn't pay and that's okay. I'm investing in my reputation, building a portfolio of writing credits. I'm still refining my voice when I'm offered a regular gig with an online MS outlet. Convinced that my mouthiness is what makes *Tripping on Air* stand out among the sugar-coated masses, I am committed to doubling down on my snarky perspective. I submit my first article, a piece about finding gratitude with chronic illness, and when the editor sends me an email with the subject "language concerns," I discover that not everyone is a fan. Could I find another word for *shitty* and reconsider the phrase *threw up in my mouth*? Even my use of the word *damn* is deemed "not to add anything in this instance."

I could take this feedback in stride, rise to the occasion and meet the challenge of coming up with a shitty synonym and a less disgusting way to describe disgust. A real writer is capable of tailoring their craft to their audience, but I resign in a huff instead. I'm not turning down the gig because I'm an asshole (though I am kind of being an asshole), I'm turning it down because I'm an *artist.* I just don't want to work on something that feels like anyone could write it. Already too big for my breeches, I realize that, just like opera singers, bloggers (writers?) can be prima donnas too.

They say write what you know, but I don't know that I want to write exclusively about MS. Maybe I want to write about food or fashion or sibling fucking rivalry. I start pitching around and land at the digital version of *xoJane* (RIP), the magazine I read from cover to cover as a teenager. *xoJane* loves my sassiness and accepts almost all of my pitches, publishing articles about tourism in Toronto, a maple syrup heist and a piece called "Bucket or Fuck It." When my first story comes out, I find fifty-four glowing comments within the first hour of its release. Only one person calls me a dick, and even that feels kind of awesome. It's not *The New Yorker* or *Vanity Fair* (yet), but if what makes a writer a writer is an enormous ego, publication and a paycheque, well, my sister can suck it, because in the spring of 2016 I receive my first-ever cheque for something I've written: fifty (US!) dollars. I have arrived.

After finding success with glorified listicles and humorous hot takes, I am ready to write a real story, something important, something journalistic. I pitch *xoJane* my most ambitious article yet: a story about beauty and disability and what I've observed as a recent mobility aid user. I want to write about the frustration of searching for young style icons who look like a cleaned-up version of me. I propose that people with disabilities shouldn't have to settle for inner-beauty bullshit—I want to write an article that proves disability can be beautiful on the outside too.

I pitch *xoJane,* telling them that "I wasn't born with a disability, but as an adult, I'm forced to create a new identity that includes it. My search for examples to inspire my acceptance of a new way of being has as much to do with how I feel about myself as it does about how others perceive me," I write. "In the absence of representation, the message can only be that disability cannot be beautiful and I'm no longer willing to accept that. Fashion is where we look to see the heightened, idealized versions of ourselves that help shape our style, which is critical to identity . . . Vanity and self-obsession are part of my North American birthright and I want back in."

xoJane says yes, write the story. And if getting paid fourteen cents a word doesn't legitimize my professionalism, I know I'm one step closer to becoming a true writer because of the procrastination cleaning I'm doing as I put off articulating what feels like a radical new idea, in 2016 at least: Disability isn't yet widely accepted as a part of diversity. Ableism is an "ism" most people have never heard of. Effectively communicating my thesis feels existentially crucial. I cannot fuck this up.

I decide to write an essay about the evolution of my personal style and how mobility aids fit into it. My closet was forced to make room for disability even before I needed to add a cane or a rollator to my looks. When I started using an ankle foot orthotic (AFO), I had to figure out if I wanted to hide my disability under a flowy skirt and a thick knee sock to keep the brace from gouging my leg or put it all out there over skinny jeans and submit to random questions about what the hell happened to me.

Either way, you can't wear heels with an AFO. When I choose safety over style, I'm restricted to flats: but not just any flats. I have to size up to Shrek shoes that include a supportive back. Open toes, mules, flip-flops and ballet flats are not options. All my shoes must have a significant tread. I could get excited about bringing back my eight-hole Doc Martens, but with drop foot—a common MS symptom that is exactly what it sounds like—they're just too heavy.

My beloved block-heeled shooties and the wine-coloured Fluevogs have to go. Both pairs are in excellent condition, and I feel like Mother Teresa for donating them instead of selling them on consignment. I can be ruthless when editing my closet, but there are certain pieces I will never part with. My fox-fur earmuffs, my raw silk turban and my 1990s embroidered denim jacket have never been out of rotation. I'm probably too old for the champagne-coloured tulle skirt I bought a decade ago, but wear it I did last Christmas. The blanket coat that kept me warm when I first got off the plane at seventeen, alone in Paris, is so faded and dated it looks absurd to me now, but every time I see it in the chest with the wool blankets, I remember the best parts of being seventeen. Like the empire-waist black satin time capsule I wore to prom, sartorial souvenirs make for more powerful memories than the madeleines I ate while wearing them. The girl, the student, the bride I was all get a place in the Ard-chives: The Museum of Every Me.

It was hard enough to part with the bulk of my shoe collection, but even Mother T wouldn't expect me to simply give away my Louboutins. It makes sense that my most storied stilettos would be retired to the vaults of my permanent collection, but I'm still not ready to stick them in the storage locker and call time of death. I'm in the denial stage of grief, clinging to the hope that I might recover enough strength and balance to one day wear them again. Which is not at all how chronic progressive illness works. I can't decide if my unwearable shoes are bullying me like a pair of too-tight aspirational jeans, holding me hostage, preventing me from accepting my body as it is, or if they're simply trying to protect me from giving in to a life of Crocs.

Before I return the shoe box to the back of my closet, I suddenly come up with an idea. I get back on my laptop and ask *xoJane* for six times as much as they normally pay me. This is not an early example of me knowing my worth as a writer—the money's not even for me. I want to hire a photographer so that my article can include images of babes with MS using a cane, a walker and a wheelchair—and yes, my Louboutins. Once again, *xoJane* agrees.

Darcy may seem like the least-appropriate beneficiary of dangerously high heels. Darcy can't walk at all. A full-time wheelchair user, Darcy's feet are mostly decorative, which I think makes them perfect for functionless shoes. She won't need to balance on skinny six-inch stems. She can sit on her throne, throw one leg over the other and let the compliments come to her. These shoes weren't made for walking, they were made to be seen. Darcy, too, deserves to be seen. So do I. So does everyone with a disability who has been left off the pages of magazines.

On the day of the photoshoot, Darcy makes the hour-long drive from her apartment in the burbs to my downtown loft in a vehicle that has been fitted with hand controls. She arrives in a new dress her dad bought her for the occasion. It's black with white polka dots and will look perfect with the red-soled stilettos. Darcy will be the article's wheelchair model, I'll be photographed with a cane, and a third model, Celia—a woman with MS who I met while being treated with alemtuzumab—will be our rollator model.

The energy in the loft is upbeat, excited, joyful. I've hired a hair and makeup artist to get us camera-ready. I put Celia in one of my favourite dresses, a swishy black mini tank dress with a scalloped hemline trimmed with white piping. I drape her in reams of pearls. When I present Darcy with the shoes likc she's Cinderella, I don't get the reaction I'm expecting.

"Ard, those shoes are never going to fit."

"Well, of course not! Nobody *fits* in a Louboutin. You cram your foot in there and accept that the price of beauty is pain," I reason. But Darcy is right. Her feet are swollen and purple from constantly sitting. There's no way we are getting her foot into that bitch of a slipper.

I am gutted. I never forgot the pain in Darcy's voice all those years ago in the parking lot of The Bean Bar, when she looked at me and practically cried, "You can wear heels?"

But Darcy is unfazed. She knew these shoes would never work and had been humouring me from the start. She pulls a pair of wide soft leather flats out of her bag. Problem solved. Move on.

When my article comes out, the response is overwhelming. I wish I could give everyone who is forced to wear their disability a confidence-boosting glow-up and a platform to see and be seen. Darcy and Celia both look gorgeous and happy. We all do. When women feel good in their skin, it's contagious, and seeing their beauty helps me see mine.

My take on representation and identity doesn't even scratch the surface of the practical concerns people with disabilities encounter when getting dressed: that clothing looks different on seated bodies, that the seams of pants can lead to pressure sores, that buttons can be enraging for anyone who lacks finger dexterity. These are just a few of the many complications I'm still learning about myself.

I decide to ditch the stilettos. They are quickly scooped up on Marketplace by a woman who doesn't even try to drive the price down. Her husband is footing the bill. He did something bad and she'd like him to feel the full consequence of his actions. I feel satisfied that the shoes have found a suitable home and a new sense of purpose.

A few weeks later, I'm still thinking about what I want to do next when I get an email from a television production executive who wants to meet me. He read my article on beauty and disability. He's creeped my blog. He wants to know if I've ever thought about making a TV show. He says, "You're a great writer." I pick up the phone and call my sister.

39 / Worst Day Ever So Far

I'M TOO OLD to be drinking watered-down gin and tonic from a plastic cup in the basement of a dive bar in New York City's Koreatown. It's not just me. Everyone crammed into the tiny, windowless room is too long in the tooth to even be up this late, a fact that's obscured by exceptionally low lighting, novelty wigs, oversized glasses and pink feather boas. Our middle-aged party of fifteen or twenty people can't party like we used to, but we're sure as hell gonna try. It's late December 2018, and The Banker and I are in town to celebrate Mike's fortieth birthday.

"Eminem. Must be Ard. You're up next," says Mike, handing me one of the two microphones our group has been provided with. COVID hasn't happened yet, so it doesn't occur to me to think about the quality of the overcrowded room's ventilation system, but my cooties radar is always on high alert for high-touch surfaces like doorknobs, elevator buttons and sweaty communal microphones. I pull down my sleeve so that my skin doesn't make contact with what I'm sure is a breeding ground of pathogens. I'm being paranoid—a party-pooper germaphobe—but it's flu season and I definitely saw Danny, who's dressed like Elton John from the waist up and is otherwise wearing only boxers, lick one of the mics during his rendition of "I Feel Love." Despite my best efforts, I've lost track of which microphone he defiled.

Mike clocks my hesitation; he's known me long enough to understand how I feel about reckless exposure to potential coughs, colds and flus. He knows what infections can do to my MS.

"Want a microphone dome?" he asks, pointing to a dusty box of thin black socks sitting on the coffee table.

"Huh, would you look at that." I'm impressed to learn that microphone condoms exist, even if they do seem kind of useless. I slip the protector over the mic and relax into my false sense of security. It's time to lose myself. It's time to party.

Danny graduates to show tunes, The Banker busts out LL Cool J, and

Mike and Lawson sing Kenny Rogers and Dolly Parton duets. Another gin and tonic and I'm officially having a blast. Just after midnight, pizza appears from I don't even know where, but I decide it's time to bounce. The closest thing to responsible adults in the room, The Banker and I are the first to leave. It's a busy weekend ahead and I need to pace myself.

The next morning, I congratulate myself on my stamina. I got on a plane and partied past midnight. I pat myself on the back for still being cool, then acknowledge my headache with a handful of Tylenol and half a litre of water.

We're in New York to celebrate Mike, but I'm just as excited to be in the Big Apple because it's Christmas. Mike insists that Manhattan in December is a fucking nightmare, but I'm more Elf than Ebenezer. I want to see the Rockefeller tree, shop at Henri Bendel (RIP again, still mourning) and sip peppermint lattes while gazing at the Fifth Avenue window displays.

"Do you want to walk first? Or do you want a push?" The Banker's talking about the mobility aid I've baptized "Optimus Prime" because of its real-life Transformer capabilities. With a few slick moves, OP converts from a rollator to a transport chair, allowing me to mitigate fatigue by walking when I'm able and getting a push when I need one. Travelling with Optimus means being able to enjoy a full day on the town instead of needing to lie down for three hours in the afternoon.

"Why don't you push me until we get to Fifth and then I can use my energy to check out the shops? No sense wasting energy on the boring parts."

The Banker's legs are long and his gait is quick. Soon, Cartier's neoclassical flagship store is within sight. Wrapped in two hundred feet of bright red ribbon and 95,000 lights, it's a six-storey Christmas present that feeds my more-is-more aesthetic. Mike isn't totally wrong about the holidays bringing out the worst of Manhattan, though. You have to be aggressive if you want to get close to the window displays, and rolling past FAO Schwarz reinforces my belief in birth control. But the seventy-two-foot tree in Rockefeller Square takes my breath away.

As we're getting ready for dinner, I receive another round of applause from The Banker for how much walking I've been able to do. *Yeah*, I think, putting on my black cashmere sweater and ostrich-feather miniskirt. *I'm fucking killing it.* The Banker's killing it too, pushing me when I need him to. *Teamwork makes the dream work.* I don't have the heart to tell him that I'm ready to collapse. I intend to rally anyway.

"We don't have to leave for half an hour. Do you want to grab a drink at the bar before dinner?" he asks.

"So badly," I reply. We're staying at the Empire, the hotel across from Lincoln Center, where *Gossip Girl* was filmed. The lobby bar is sexy and moody and made for selfies. "But I think I should take advantage of the chance to sneak in a rest. Also, do we have any more Tylenol?" My throat is dry and I blame airplane air and karaoke. Too many gin and tonics and not enough water. I prop myself on the bed with enough pillows behind my back that I can stretch out my legs without compromising my hair. I tell myself that thirty minutes off my feet will be enough to revive me.

When it's time to leave, I'm a little anxious that my brief rest and acetaminophen appetizer didn't exactly have the effect of speed or even caffeine. I also can't seem to warm up, so I slip a throw blanket from the hotel room into the bag attached to the back of Optimus.

We're meeting Mike and Co. at Keens Steakhouse, a New York City institution. The vibe is a one-eighty from the black-lit, barely concealed STD scene of the previous night's festivities. Keens is a grown-up restaurant. Keens is your dad's restaurant. It's been around since the late 1800s and has a pipe room—whatever that means. It has enough male energy that I make a note to google how long they've been letting women dine there. (Answer: not at all, until there was a lawsuit.)

The restaurant isn't entirely accessible, but I'm so used to finding workarounds, because almost nothing is. The dining room is sunken, down three or four steps. Annoying, but manageable, even with my fatigue, and at least it's on the same floor as the bathroom. I grab my cane while The Banker tucks OP in a corner and a waiter lends me his arm to help me down the stairs. We're the last to arrive, and Mike's at the opposite end of the long table, holding court, already tipsy. I'm sitting next to Danny, the microphone licker, who's actually growing on me with his loud personality and even louder wardrobe. New York is the first place Danny—a gay kid from the South—feels like he can be his shiny gay self.

Danny has decided we're best friends now and helps himself to a sip of my Manhattan. *Great, there goes my twenty-five-dollar cocktail.* A real best friend would know I do not swap saliva. I take a sip of water in silent protest and that's when I realize that my throat isn't just dry, it's for sure sore. I don't know what germs Danny's packing, but it's too late to tell him he might have just sipped some contagions of my own.

I don't blame Eminem, or airplane air. Karaoke is the adult equivalent of hanging out in the ball pit at Chuck E. Cheese—a cesspool of risk—but it was only twenty-four hours ago. Whatever bug I'm fighting has been incubating since Canada. This bug is imported.

I start to plan my escape. I contemplate finishing my con*Dan*imated Manhattan, telling myself that you can't get more than one thing at a time, telling myself that the alcohol will kill some of the germs at the back of my throat. *Fuck it; I've already lost the battle.* I swallow what's left in one gulp. It hurts enough that I'm not interested in sticking around long enough to try the cheesecake.

I brief The Banker discreetly. I want to slip out without causing a scene. Mike is reasonably drunk and distracted. I'll text him later. The Banker goes to get Optimus, but when I try to stand up it's like my weight has doubled. The stairs I'd negotiated with a cane and the arm of an anonymous man are suddenly impossible. In the span of a few hours I've gone from prancing around the city, shopping and posing for pics, to "I can't fucking stand up." I guess I live in the basement of a haunted steakhouse now.

The Banker pulls out his best can-do attitude. He helps me slide from the leather dining room chair and onto Optimus Prime. Before I can worry about what happens next, I'm suddenly in the air. The Banker and the waiter are carrying me up the stairs in my transport chair. I half-expect the theme song from *Chariots of Fire* to start playing. So much for not making a scene.

I have a rush of emotions. FOMO. Dismay. Guilt over what The Banker is going to miss, anger at what I have let happen to myself. But my biggest feeling is fear. Yeah, I might have a cold, I might even have the flu, but worse than both of those things is the possibility that I'm having a pseudo-relapse.

Pseudo-relapses can be caused by increases in body temperature from fever, or exercise, or a butterfly flapping its wings. These relapse fake-outs resolve with rest and a return to regular body temperature. But when infections prompt the immune system to produce cytokines, pseudo-relapses can have more serious implications. Satan's cytokine envoy travels to the brain to provoke a bar fight with the microglia, or injury-repair cells. A pseudo-relapse can reactivate symptoms that have resolved, or make existing symptoms worse. A pseudo-relapse may even trigger an actual relapse. The possibility of not recovering back to baseline or accelerating MS progression is what makes colds and flus such a potential freaking nightmare for people with MS.

Outside, it's cold and dark and drizzly. Our home base is a thirty-minute walk away, but I can't physically get out of my chair to get into a cab. So we walk. I mean, The Banker walks. Practically jogs. Pushing me in my transport chair. I sit wrapped and shivering in the hotel blanket, feeling defeated and small.

By the time we get back to the hotel, I can't sit up on my own. I'm shaking uncontrollably. We don't need a thermometer to know that I have a raging fever. The Banker wraps his whole body around me to keep me warm, holding me tight.

I spend the next twenty-four hours trying on what it feels like to have to ask for help for Every. Single. Thing. I feel demoralized by my constant "pleases" and "thank yous" for things I never wanted to need. A glass of water, a trip to the bathroom, help just to sit up. I'm entirely dependent on my partner. (Are we still partners if this is our relationship dynamic?)

With enough time and Tylenol, my temperature returns to its reptilian baseline. As I recover, I'm relieved to find I can once again get to the bathroom by myself. But it's not an "all's well that ends well" kind of story. My walking isn't nearly as strong as it was a week ago, and I don't know if it ever will be. My pseudo-relapse showed me what my MS could look like when my reserve capacity runs out; it gave me a taste of where my MS progression is headed. Like a real-life visit from a dark Dickensian ghost, for a few days this Christmas I had a glimpse of a future that feels more inevitable than ever, and it's terrifying. I guess I'm more Ebenezer than Elf after all.

40 / Hard to Swallow

"ARDY, ARE YOU SICK? It sounds like there's a frog in your throat," my brother asks over the phone.

"No, impossible," I answer. I don't feel sick, plus there's no way I've been exposed to germs. It's early COVID Times and The Banker and I haven't stepped outside our two-person bubble. At all. I haven't even left the apartment in weeks. Whatever's going on with my voice is coming from inside the house. BRB, I have to ask Google if "Apartment Lung" is a thing.

I'm not exactly sure when this frog took up residence in my throat anyway. Has it been days? Weeks? It's hard to tell, because the croaking seems to come and go. Suddenly, and for no apparent reason, the frog shows up and my voice gets thin and raspy. Not in the familiar post–respiratory infection laryngitis way, or even the morning-after-a-night-of-loud-talking-and-drinking way, but in an entirely new and confounding way. When I open my mouth to speak, what comes out doesn't match my expectations. Instead of sounding clear and confident like my loud loquacious self, I sound like Marge's mom on *The Simpsons*. Old and weary. The simple act of talking sucks the energy out of me. It's like my speech gets fatigued the same way my everything-else does.

And there's the red flag.

I've been trying to convince myself that my sudden speech problem isn't a problem. I probably just need a nap, but James's question means that the frog isn't in my head—whatever's going on is noticeable. Real.

I'm convinced that MS is the cause of all my body's fuckery but the fact that MS could impact my vocal quality beyond the effects of fatigue and lack of stamina is barely on my radar. I follow Dr. Google down a rabbit hole and learn that if Kermit is indeed caused by MS, his real name is Dysarthria. I don't know anyone with MS who has dysarthria and so the symptom feels unlikely and rare—like white peacocks, or Starbucks getting my name right. I assume dysarthria is one of those late-stage symptoms of advanced MS: theoretical and not something I need to worry about. At least not for a long time.

I'm ready to close this browser and see what's on sale at Sephora—but Dr. Google isn't done with me yet.

"Psst. Ardra. Have you thought about dysphagia?"

"No . . ."

I reluctantly keep reading and discover that dysphagia is the medical term for difficulty swallowing. People with dysarthria might also have dysphagia. I take a hypochondriac pause to consider the scene I made on Monday when my gin martini decided to take the road less travelled. (Martini Mondays are a thing for us now because, again, The Banker and I are riding out quarantine in a one-bedroom apartment, and it's easier to tell what day it is by assigning fun alliterative drinks.) When I tried to coax my errant cocktail out of my lungs it was like my body forgot how to cough. All I could do was flail my arms and make a pathetic *a-heh* sound.

"Oh yeah, dysphagia can impair the coughing reflex," Dr. Google volunteers.

"And what happens if you get gin in your lungs? Is that a big deal? Is Gin Lung a thing?"

Bacteria can enter the lungs and cause infections like aspirational pneumonia, I read.

Well, that's a fucked-up thing to call it. I do not aspire to pneumonia. We're done here. I slam my laptop shut.

It's Whisky Wednesday and I, for one, could use a drink. I decide to kill two birds and do some science on myself by paying closer attention to how my next beverage goes down. I know I'm being ridiculous. I can't have dysphagia any more than I can have dysarthria. Even more than dysarthria, dysphagia definitely feels like a late-stage symptom. Probably because it can kill you. *She died of causes related to MS. Choking on a martini.*

Nevertheless, my speech and swallowing seem to get worse over the coming days and weeks. I gag on water and no longer feel safe eating anything in the shredded food group. And fine, I can live without tacos, but it's hard not to stress over what a future without talking looks like. The Banker and I have only moderate-grade marital ESP. Our non-verbal communication is mostly limited to looks that mean *Save me, I don't know this dude's name* and *If you eat the rest of the chips, we will have a problem*. If The Banker is forced to carry our conversations I will die from exposure to small talk.

Without words I will be left with eye rolls and resting bitch face for casual communication, and I've got so much more to say. I don't use my voice only for gossip and complaining: lately I've been covering the French portion of my niece's pandemic-induced home-schooling. I don't sing much anymore, but I'd like to have the option.

I don't know why I feel the need to articulate how much it would suck to lose speech. I've spent my life talking, and maybe that's the problem. I've used up my allotment.

I call the MS clinic, but again, COVID Times means it's gonna take a while to get some answers. In an added twist of frustration, the new drug I'm supposed to start—the one that might have prevented this new symptom, if that's what it is—is immunosuppressive. I will have to delay treatment until after I can have the necessary diagnostics since nobody wants to send me into the hospital in the middle of a pandemic with less than all my defences.

I ride out this latest period of purgatory trying to avoid talking while eating. I start chewing my food with conscious conviction like every bite is one of those smug-ass meditation raisins. I use what I know about breath and singing to try and power my speech.

After I finally get an appointment with the MS clinic, I check my MRI results online as soon as they're available. The images mean nothing to me, and I skip right to the findings. "There is a large new intramedullary lesion within the left lateral medulla." This shouldn't be shocking, but it is. Instead of taking the news in stride, I burst into tears, like a rookie. In the hierarchy of MS symptoms, new ones are a chilling reminder that despite all my interventions, MS is always lurking, waiting to fuck shit up.

I'm angry. New lesions aren't supposed to happen to me. And that's not hubris talking—at least it's not *my* hubris: I was told I didn't need to be on meds, that I was secondary progressive and that my disease was stable. MS isn't like other conditions that have obvious consensus-based treatment plans. There's no "take this drug or you will die" clarity. Doctors have vastly different opinions. *If only I'd had treatment X a little earlier* is a heartbreaking path I've been down all too often. But this doesn't feel like heartbreak. Knowing that if I'd been given the drug I begged for—which might have prevented this relapse—fuels a rage that is hard to articulate. This didn't have to happen, though I am expected to take it in stride. *These things happen.*

The work of adapting begins with a speech pathologist. I spend my precious energy learning about things like thickened water and safe swallowing techniques, then decide that I'd rather roll the dice on my new and potentially life-threatening symptom than add a thickening agent to Tequila Tuesdays. I'm told to keep the inside of my mouth as clean as possible so that if I do choke, at least it will be on something less germy. I invest in an electric toothbrush. I practise basic breathing and reading out loud, trying to get one sentence out in one breath, and feel the long-ago but familiar frustration of grade-school group reading time, except now the slow kid is me.

I resent how much work I have to do, just trying to catch up to who I used to be. How many times will I be forced to slap on a smile, grieve and get on with it, pivot and reinvent?

As many times as it takes, I guess.

41 / Number-One Problem

"I JUST LOVE THAT GLOSS," my mother-in-law gushes as I swipe a sheer plum-coloured Juicy Tube across my lips. Jan and I are standing in the parking lot, admiring each other's outfits while we wait for her son, my husband, to pay the bill and extricate himself from whatever conversation he's gotten himself into. We've had a nice visit and a decent dinner, but my MIL and I are both tired, and ready to go home. Unfortunately, The Banker is in Classic Banker Mode and is delaying our exit. Small talk is his jam.

Jan and I are putting in time, but we aren't making small talk when we chat about makeup. Fashion and beauty are subjects we both take seriously. Our styles are different—I like a bit of whimsy and a high hemline; Jan wears only trousers or jeans and thinks long hair is stupid. We both love accessories, though Jan's passion borders on actual obsession. My mother-in-law would be unrecognizable without her trinkets. Her collection of baubles prizes quantity over quality. Colour and size trump subtlety; coordination is the hallmark of her style. More Iris Apfel than Chanel, Jan is the antithesis to Coco's "take one thing off before you leave the house" aesthetic.

"I'll bring you one of these glosses next week," I tell Jan as The Banker finally emerges from the restaurant.

"It's a really great business you've got here," TB blah-blah-blahs to the owner, who has decided to see him out. The food is fine, but we were the evening's only customers, presumably because of this dead-zone location, not far from Jan's bungalow in the middle of suburban nowhere. She moved here a few years after her husband, TB's father, died.

"See you next week," I say, with a let's-get-out-of-here nod to Jan, as I start walking to the car. Too bad I'm about to unwittingly sabotage our escape. As I start to leave, I lose my balance and fall backwards off the curb. I land on my back, and then my head, smacking my skull on the concrete.

"Oh dear, oh no, oh dear," says Jan.

"I'm okay." At least I think I am. It takes a beat for me to figure out if I'm hurt or if I'm *hurt* hurt.

"Can we get a towel or something?" The Banker tries to sound calm as he inspects my injury.

"Am I bleeding?"

"Uhm . . ."

Well, that means yes. TB helps me to my feet and we decide I should probably go to the hospital. I can walk, so there's no need to call an ambulance. Jan takes the front seat and I sit in the back, holding a bag of ice wrapped in a bloodstained tea towel to the back of my throbbing head. I might be concussed, and I probably need stitches, but it's still easier for me to crawl into the back of our compact car than it is for my aging mother-in-law, whose own falls have led to her ever-increasing frailty.

"Are we going straight to the hospital?" Jan asks when we don't turn left on our way out of the parking lot. Her tone implies that she'd prefer another option.

"Of course!" The Banker says. "She's bleeding!"

My mother-in-law is generally incapable of saying what she actually means, and a few minutes later she pipes up again: "Are we dropping Ardra off or are we going to wait with her?"

The Banker grips the steering wheel. He's not great with using his words either, and the worm-like vein at his temple is so pronounced that I'm pretty sure it's become sentient.

"It's okay," I say, because, concussed or not, I don't need all my faculties to read the situation. Jan is anxious and uncomfortable and it has nothing to do with me. Jan doesn't just *want* to get home, she *needs* to get home. On some psychic, sympathetic level, I can tell that she's concerned about being close to a bathroom—that she's in the midst of her own kind of emergency. It's hard to give a shit about anything else if you think you might poop your pants.

I have some awareness of how aging impacts the bowels. Jan doesn't talk about her body's betrayal but I've picked up the clues, and seen enough evidence to know. Generally, I try to help discreetly, making her Metamucil-tinis at Happy Hour (two parts water, one part prune juice, mix vigorously with psyllium fibre, serve in a chilled martini glass). I've been ordering her groceries ever since she stopped driving, slipping in items that she doesn't ask for but never objects to, like Poise pads and Depends, onto her weekly list of essentials (root beer, cottage cheese, hot dogs, grapes, *People* magazine, the orange juice that's easy to open).

It's not like Jan to discuss the scatological. She doesn't have a potty mouth—Jan is a *lady.* The potential for humiliation might be part of what compels my mother-in-law to suffer in silence, but until she was widowed, Jan spent forty years answering to someone else. Now, in the absence of anyone telling her what to eat, who to see, where to go and how to get there, Jan is forced to figure out what she really wants (a leather jacket, a date with the minister, celebrity gossip, reality TV), but she still isn't comfortable with self-advocacy. My MIL smiles and laughs easily now (well, not right now), but I didn't always know this version of her. For years, she would sit silently in the corner at family gatherings, arms folded across her chest, while her husband held court. Beyond her low-simmering resentment, the only hint of her true identity was her expertly applied makeup, tailored outfit and, most essentially, her carefully coordinated accessories.

I can't expect a woman with this kind of history, let alone commitment to her own image, to talk openly about incontinence. I'm no introvert, and I always say what I mean, but even as a professional over-sharer, I am loathe to talk about my own scatological stuff. In the language of my WASPy grandmother who, like my husband and MIL, also refused to call anything like it is, my problem with number two is often my number-one problem.

I am all too familiar with prayers uttered in vain to indifferent deities: *Hail Mary, full of grace, please don't let me die of humiliation. Wait, scratch that. Holy Mary, mother of God, in thy mercy, smite me dead so that I don't have to suffer this humiliation.*

Not surprisingly, the Blessed Virgin almost always has better things to concern herself with than my wounded dignity. I'm on my own. And frankly, that's how I want it. Let me hide in the bathroom for two hours in peace.

Jan and I are both in distress while The Banker is tasked with trying to suss out which one of us requires the most urgent attention. Neither of us is in a life-threatening situation. Even if you want to die, technically, bowel incontinence won't kill you. (Well, not directly. If you're already a falls risk, running to the restroom when you can't actually run can be a recipe for disaster. Worse if the washroom is down a flight of stairs.) But there's minimal blood coming out of my head, and I can tell my injury isn't going to end me either. I can wait alone to get a few stitches, so I throw my support behind Jan.

"Drop me at urgent care, then take your mom home and come back for me. I'll probably still be in triage," I say. The Banker opens his mouth to protest but I catch his eye in the rear-view mirror. "It's fine," I say. "Trust me."

SIX YEARS LATER, Jan still sucks at asking for help. Meanwhile, her recently discovered self is being eroded in long-term care. She doesn't get to choose who she sits next to at dinner, let alone what she gets to eat. Once again she is reduced to self-expression by way of costume jewellery. Her collection has been edited with the ruthlessness of Marie Kondo, from dresser drawers overflowing with knots of chunky acrylic and a cartoon pirate's treasure chest distilled into a few dozen pieces.

Long-term care is circle nine and a half of hell, where UTIs flourish and under-resourced staff leave residents ("inmates," according to Jan) sitting in diapers. When Jan's PSW can't be bothered to help her draw her eyebrows straight, I try to find Jan a lipstick or suggest a necklace and some earrings to help her feel like herself.

Our broken health-care system is as enraging as it is terrifying, and because I make everything about me, I worry about one day ending up in uncaring long-term care myself. For one thing, I did not spend my life cultivating a palate for cheese that smells like cabbage to end up eating Kraft slices and sheet cake on special occasions. There are plenty of reasons to find long-term care unappealing, and I consider developing a cat allergy in an effort to keep myself off the guest list. The only redeeming quality of long-term care facilities is that they tend to be heated to my satisfaction. But a thermostat set to twenty-eight degrees Celsius is not enough for me to get past my total lack of confidence in how these places manage bladder and bowel function.

I still don't have my shit together—in fact, my neurogenic bowel seems to be getting worse lately. But the Virgin Mary works in mysterious ways, and COVID lockdowns are making it easier for me to manage in a less disruptive way. I don't have to explain why I prefer to start my workday at whenever-the-fuck-my-MS-feels-like-it o'clock. That one of my first experiences in a real-life writers' room is happening remotely is less of a bummer because it lets me deal with my bum.

Morning routines are trending, and social media is filled with scenes of sunrises, yoga and espresso-based coffees: Me Time that doesn't exist in the MS Time Zone. My morning relies on a decidedly less Instagrammable calculation of suppositories, supplements, laxatives and patience that results in only a "fingers crossed" situation more than anything resembling a guarantee. Anyone who claims "I have MS, but MS doesn't have me" has escaped bladder and bowel dysfunction, or else refuses to consider how bathroom routines can feel like MS has you by the ass.

Anyway, The Banker is banking from home when, first thing Monday morning, the phone rings. It's the doctor (well, *a* doctor) with an update on Jan's latest UTI. Infections exacerbate Jan's Lewy body dementia, and when Jan is confused, isn't herself or has a sudden change in cognitive function, we've gotten in the habit of insisting on a urine test. If I were in charge of long-term care, every bathroom would have a bidet.

I slide over to TB's desk and he puts the call on speaker. "I've been wondering about your mother's UTIs and whether or not they've all been UTIs or if this is just the natural progression of her disease," the doctor, who doesn't even know Jan, says. "I suppose the question is whether we want to send her to the hospital or focus on making her comfortable."

What? Wouldn't some antibiotics make her comfortable? The Banker and I look at each other, the same just-been-slapped expression of confusion on our faces. We both know UTIs can be life-threatening, but only because they can lead to kidney infections and sepsis. I put my hand on my husband's knee before asking the doctor what feels like a ludicrous question. "Are you saying she's palliative?!"

He is. Or I guess I am. Doctors have a way of making you name the terrible thing yourself. Like bad boyfriends who, instead of breaking up with you, sulk and act distant. They wait for you to realize what they refuse to say themselves, until the moment of their exoneration when, with a furrowed brow, the question "Wait, are you breaking up with me?" dawns on their gaslit girlfriends' faces.

"How did it come to this? What is happening now?" I ask.

"She's confused, as you noted; she's also refusing to eat."

I bristle at the word *refusing*. This is a medical issue—she's not being petulant. "What exactly does keeping her comfortable mean?"

"Morphine, oxygen, anxiety meds."

"If she's not eating, does this plan include fluids?" It does not. I ask about the pain of death by starvation and dehydration, and am told there's no evidence this process is painful. Why the morphine then?

We end the call and try to process the intel.

"Pros: if we send her to the hospital, she might pull through with antibiotics," I open.

"Cons: the last time she went to the hospital for one thing she came out with something else. If there's another COVID outbreak, she could be stuck there for months," TB counters.

"Cons: there's always another outbreak."

"Cons: there's always another UTI."

"Cons: she can only have one visitor for one hour a day."

"Cons: if I go to the hospital to see her, I could be exposing you to COVID."

"Cons: if she goes to the hospital, there's a chance she could die alone."

Cons. Cons. Cons.

"Your mom hasn't seen you for months because of the lockdowns. She hasn't been touched by anyone she loves. The doctor said palliative patients in long-term care are allowed unlimited time with immediate family members. I think we need to redefine the 'pros.'"

The Banker and his brother spend the next week taking shifts at their mother's bedside. Jan sleeps a lot, but when she's awake, she's with it. She tries to talk and sometimes she succeeds.

TB FaceTimes me from her room, though I can barely see his face. He's in full PPE and he looks like the feds from the movie *E.T.* Jan knows she's dying, and TB cycles between sentimental support and trying to lighten the mood. Each day he brings an armful of the heavy scrapbooks I've made that document our life together over the past seventeen years. When Jan can't open her eyes, he describes every picture in detail. She smiles when he asks where she buried the gold, the twinkle still in her eye. He plays music, holds her hand, rubs her feet, sings, dances, tells her he loves her. When he wonders if she'd like to punch God in the face, she mouths, "Yes," and punches the air. When he uses a damp cloth to moisten his mother's lips, he tells her he wishes it were lipstick.

"I don't care about lipstick," she manages to say, before quickly issuing a retraction. "Yes, I do."

The phone wakes us at 5 a.m. Thanksgiving Sunday. Good news never comes in the wee hours before sunrise. No ring tone exists that can make a 5 a.m. phone call sound anything other than ominous. Sure enough, there have been dramatic changes to Jan's breathing. It's time to go.

COVID restrictions prevent me from saying goodbye to Jan in person. Only her sons are allowed to see her. But I should be in the car for the drive, waiting with the dog—TB shouldn't have to do this alone. Of course, I'm not going anywhere, because I'm tethered to my morning routine, a plan that was set in motion at least eighteen hours ago. MS doesn't make room for spontaneity, never mind early morning emergencies. Trapped in this body, the reason I am not in the car with my husband on this heartbreaking day is as simple (and as complicated) as not being able to trust my bowel. How ridiculous. I feel useless. It doesn't matter that this is a medical issue, and not a failure of my character. I feel like I'm failing at Wife.

At 9:30 a.m., TB texts to tell me his mother is gone. This is not a day to feel sorry for myself. It's time to get my shit together. The Banker is always the first to point out that we support each other in different ways, according to our unique gifts and abilities. I can't go back in time and un-fuck my bowel, but I can take comfort in the hours I poured into the scrapbooks that served as my surrogate, my contribution to the process of remembering, of saying goodbye. I know TB doesn't feel like I failed him today, and I know Jan, of all people, would get it.

I can also put into words, into memory, the details of how a son kept vigil at his mother's bedside and made sure she had a good death. I can articulate the fuzzy details he may already have forgotten, and remind him of the time when the world was in chaos, nothing was normal—or would ever be normal again—and still, somehow, he was able to be the best version of himself.

42 / Patient Days

ONCE UPON A TIME, a curious massage therapist asked me what I do all day.

"So, do you just, like, watch TV?" he asked. Granted, this question came from a *student* therapist, a kid who was probably no more than twenty-one.

"Sure, TV," I said, face down on the massage table, hoping he could hear me rolling my eyes. I wasn't about to explain myself, but it's also way less mortifying to cop to watching TV all day than it is to say, "Actually, I'm a blogger. I take selfies and talk smack on the internet."

My take on day-in-the-life questions is that they are tedious at best, and, if I'm feeling cynical—which I almost always am—they're veiled accusations. When people ask me what I do all day, I suspect it's because they lack the imagination to think I can do anything at all, or they think I'm living the lazy-girl dream, living off the system.

Except for Patient Days, chances are I'm doing the same mundane activities as everyone else: a little eating, basic grooming, looking at screens, avoiding phone calls, ordering from Amazon and petting some dogs, if I'm lucky.

Today happens to be a Patient Day and The Banker has rearranged his schedule so that he can drive me to the hospital. I'm not sick, at least not acutely. Probably. I'm on immunosuppressive drugs, so there's always a chance I'm harbouring some yet-to-be-detected infection. The risk of undiscovered issues is compounded by years of chronic pain that have trained me not to listen to my constantly complaining body. Nerve pain is a mind-fuck and tuning it out is a survival strategy. At least until I die of sepsis, or rabies, or dysentery, after confusing general malaise with the life-threatening kind.

A negligence-induced death is a problem for Future Me. Today I'm at North York General, because chronic illness means that even on a good day you might find me at any number of medical facilities in the Greater Toronto Area. Having MS means having Patient Days.

Patient Days can include doctors, appointments, infusions, lab work, X-rays, bone scans, MRIs and other medical tests. Patient Days involve paperwork, phone calls, physio, insurance claims—basically any activity that's part of the business of having a disease. Patient Days are the unpaid labour of keeping myself alive. You know, when I'm not watching TV.

At best, Patient Days are an inconvenient time-sucking, energy-sucking, money-sucking—and, once a month or so, literal blood-sucking—reality of life with MS. When I was first diagnosed, Patient Days could be traumatizing. MRIs were scary and spinal taps were worse. Like a kid being bribed with a lollipop, when Patient Days were difficult, I would reward myself. Bruised from a blood draw? That's worth a latte. A call from insurance merits a mid-week cocktail—assuming the call went to voice mail. Having to talk to an actual agent nets a cashmere sweater. Leaky spinal fluid after a half-assed lumbar puncture? That's a trip to France.

Along with the costs of things like transportation and time off work, my increasingly sophisticated reward system eventually became untenable. With too much trauma for my budget to soothe, my pain tolerance had to evolve. I learned how to mostly take Patient Days in stride. Now I tell myself I can do hard things, then go through the motions, trying not to dwell on the fact that Patient Days are a routine reminder that I'm going to be sick forever.

I'm running late to my CT scan, without doing any actual running. In fact, I'm moving so slowly that no one watching would suspect I'm in a hurry. (You may be thinking, *Wait a sec, CT scan? That's not a regular part of MS monitoring!* Guess what, bitches. If you have one disease, you're more likely to get another, and another one after that!)

I have to pee, which adds ten minutes to my ETA, because it takes at least ten minutes for me to deal with buttons, and zippers, and doors, and caths; and, if I think too long about what else I could do with the approximately eighty minutes a day I need to dedicate to bladder emptying, the waste becomes overwhelming. (Also, the answer is obviously TV.)

There are no signs telling me where to find the CT department. This isn't my usual hospital, but I've been here once or twice and I sort of remember where to go.

When I'm finally in the homestretch of what feels like my four-thousand-mile trek to Imaging, there must be an urgency in my eyes because someone—a man—notices my slow walk and decides to intervene.

"Do you want a push?" he asks. This is a pretty fucked-up question, and even though it isn't ha-ha funny, I assume he's joking, because there's nothing to push. I'm not using a wheelchair—I'm walking with my rollator.

"Uh, no?" I say, feeling kind of stupid for even answering such an absurd question. But I am not the stupid person in the room, and to my horror, I suddenly feel a hand on the small of my back. This guy is actually pushing me, trying to make me go faster. Like I just need a little shove to get going.

"Please don't push me!" I say, with alarm, because his help isn't helping. It's destabilizing. Unsafe. The Pusher quickly retreats and is gone so fast I don't see where he went; and now I get to feel bad about making *him* feel bad, because he was just trying to help.

When I finally arrive at Imaging, I'm breathless. I try to balance against the reception desk so that I can fish my health card out of my bag without falling over. Before I can apologize for my tardiness, the man behind the glass window says, "Registration's back that way."

FML. I look back over my shoulder to see an identical desk an impossible thirty feet away.

I don't have the energy to protest, or even plead my case. Hospitals have trained us to be meek and apologetic just for being there, for bothering the busy staff, who are not there to make Patient Days easier but to remind you that you are an inconvenience. I forget which circle of *Inferno* Dante dedicated to hospital waiting rooms, because I never read it, but I'm pretty sure it's the job of Admin to make the experience unpleasant enough that you will eventually start asking yourself if the bleeding really is *that* bad.

As I start to make my way back to Registration, the receptionist reconsiders when he sees how pathetically I'm moving. If that motherfucker asks me if I need a push—

"Never mind. I'll check you in here," he says, taking pity on me.

Hallelujah. Good people exist. Ignore everything I just said. God bless hospital admin.

The hallway next to the waiting room is filled with people on stretchers who seem to be actively dying. There's coughing so thick with phlegm that I cannot comfort myself with the fact that I'm masked and the lie that these are the coughs of smokers and not of people spewing deadly contagions. I hear beeping, and paging, and a baby crying. Most disturbingly, an older woman who's all alone pleads, "Toilet, toillllllet," over and over. Everyone ignores her.

Finally, a nurse tells me it's time to start my IV, and even though the waiting room does indeed have a TV, I can't get out of there fast enough.

"Take your time," she says, as if I have a choice (or need her permission). She doesn't physically push me, but she watches me with an intensity that says *hurry the fuck up*, like she's psychically trying to compel me to move more quickly. This is the go-faster vibe I'm more familiar with. It's standard behaviour when getting in and out of Ubers.

"Shoot," says the nurse trying to find my vein. I don't ask. I don't even look, but I feel the trickle of blood running down my arm. In the past this kind of mishap might have led me to buy myself a new pair of earrings. Now I make a mental note to take an iron supplement later.

"No worries!" I say, prioritizing her comfort over my own, but also operating under the theory that the more nervous the nurse is, the more likely I am to bleed out before she can get an IV started.

At this point, I'm happy that a CT scan is a lying-down activity. Lying down is its own reward. I make the best of the experience by asking for a blanket.

"You might feel a warm sensation when the contrast dye is injected," the technician tells me, and to be honest, "warm sensation" also sounds kind of nice.

"Some people say it feels like they're peeing? But don't worry, you're not actually peeing." Oh.

When the contrast dye is injected, I feel it in places I didn't know I could feel things. My organs are suddenly hot and burny. *Is that my pancreas? Hello, gallbladder!* The warm sensation is more of a light toxic searing and I am one million percent certain that I am actually peeing. (I am not.)

When the exam is over, there's a smear of blood on my arm where the nurse not so much cleaned it off as . . . moved it around. I am so ready to go home and watch TV.

When I emerge from the bathroom, fully dressed and washed of arm blood, the nurse who caused the leak is waiting for me. She has a wheelchair to take me to the exit, so that I don't have to walk. I didn't ask for this help, but I realize I need it. Once again, I am grateful.

This wasn't a particularly remarkable Patient Day, but a standard mix of bureaucracy, mediocracy, idiocy—and yes—even kindness. On our way out, I make eye contact with the old lady who is still crying, "Toilet, toillllllet." I wonder how long it will take for someone to help her. I try not to wonder how long it will take for me to be her.

43 / Pride?

TOO MUCH OF THE CALENDAR is dedicated to awareness campaigns. It's getting ridiculous. We don't need Poison Prevention Week when there's a skull and crossbones on every box of poison. Cerebrospinal Fluid Leak Awareness could have been covered in an email. Meanwhile, World Rabies Day is just confusing. It's not Rabies Prevention Day or even Rabies Awareness Day. Just Rabies Day! You decide if rabies is good or bad.

Some major diseases get an entire month of awareness. Lupus even gets two: May and October. That's sixty days, every year, and still nobody knows anything reliable about lupus. I assume Radon Action Month is a time to celebrate Spider-Man's birthday, as well as an invitation to explore the potential for your own superhero origin story, but I can't be sure because awareness campaigns don't seem to do anything to actually increase awareness. If the Ice Bucket Challenge taught us anything, it's that we learned nothing about ALS from the Ice Bucket Challenge.

Even so, awareness events and races, easily identified by itchy, low-quality, disease-branded T-shirts, unlimited orange drink and the suffix *a-thon*, are powerful and meaningful events for many people. The MS Walk, *par exemple*, can be a community-building, feel-good street party of love and support. I donate to the walk every year and solicit funds on years when I get around to it, but the truth is, this event is not for me. I'm not a fan.

That I don't care for the MS Walk feels like a dirty secret, like I'm a bad MS patient, a traitor to my people and an ingrate to the organization dedicated to "finding the cure." One of the burdens of this crappy disease is the feeling that I've unwittingly agreed to a lifetime of soliciting donations from friends, family and every loose social-media contact I have. To me, awareness months feel less like celebrations of the communities they represent and more like obligations to generate pity in exchange for cash.

My first MS Walk was a stress-fest. It was scary to see people more disabled than me. I felt icky being the subject of the cheerleading teams' encouraging slogans. Seeing my name on the bibs of my friends and family, next to the words *I'm Walking for . . .* was an uncomfortable way to be the centre of attention. The money we were raising would benefit me indirectly, maybe someday, in ways that felt intangible and hard to appreciate at the time.

Over the years, I half-assed my way through these events because there are amazing people in my life who were keen to support me, and rejecting the MS Walk would have felt like a rejection of love. Eventually, my inability to walk five kilometres gave me the excuse I needed to sit things out.

Of course, the obligation to do my part didn't end when I abandoned the walk-a-thon. In 2019, the same organization asked me to go to Union Station in downtown Toronto at rush hour on World MS Day. The campaign was called Acts of Greatness, and if you're thinking Malala Yousafzai or Oskar Schindler's ghost were also invited, prepare to be disappointed.

The act of greatness I was asked to perform at this disability circus was to walk across a five-metre-long decal that read "For Canadians with mobility issues, just 5 metres can feel like 500." My struggle would be broadcast on social media, where I would then be tasked to explain my misfortune and ask strangers to text a ten-dollar donation. #ActsofGreatness.

I declined the invitation, saying that the logistics of navigating the train station were too much. This was true, but I regret not explaining how offensive this idea was to begin with. *Exploited* is a strong word, but I was unwilling to make my Inspiration Porn debut. Especially for only ten bucks an ask.

I'm better at pointing out the flaws in sketchy advocacy now. I understand that sparing feelings and trying to be polite do nothing to advance our common objective of improving the lives of people with MS. This particular organization really does care about the MS community, and in the ensuing years I have volunteered in other ways, sharing my ideas and perspective. I'm proud of the work we've done together and I appreciate the organization's receptivity to evolving with the times. I'm still not going to do the walk, but I will double my donation this year in an attempt to make amends for crapping on it in a book.

A year after my refusal to be an act of greatness, I'm leaning into my mediocrity when I become aware of Disability Pride Month. Naturally, my first reaction is suspicion. Disability Pride sounds as absurd as Sun Awareness Month (for anyone who has yet to encounter the sun). Nonetheless, I do some googling and discover that disability pride celebrations have officially been around since 1990 (at least in the US), when the Americans with Disabilities Act was signed into law. There's even a parade. Not that a parade makes the concept more appealing. The only thing worse than marching is watching other people march. I'm not putting on sunscreen to watch a two-hour traffic jam whose soundtrack is a shitty high-school band. There's a reason parades are free.

I can sit out the parade—I know my rights. Plus, of all the identities I have and am proud of, it feels messed up to throw a party for this one. I don't personally believe that disability is a fate worse than death, but plenty of other people do, and it's hard to reconcile the years of having society tell me to overcome, to fight, to not let MS define me—effectively denying my disability—then turn around and tell me to feel proud. I'm confused.

Disabled was (and continues to be) an excruciatingly difficult identity for me to accept. The thought of attaching the word *pride* to the thing that diminishes me, that literally brings me to my knees (and bum, and the floor), is an idea I choke on. Disabled is the thing that everyone is afraid of becoming. Disabled doesn't feel like something to celebrate.

Still, I feel like I owe it to my disabled peers to try and figure it out. My discovery of Disability Pride Month coincides with the release of the Netflix documentary *Crip Camp,* which I decide to watch. It's about a summer camp in the Catskills where disabled teens in the early 1970s were allowed to be teens like everyone else. The kids played sports, smoked pot and even hooked up. Nobody had considered that they were sexual beings, as horny and reckless as their non-disabled peers. As camper Denise Sherer Jacobson says in the film, "My doctor came in, and he gave me a pelvic exam and said, 'You know . . . I think you might have gonorrhea.' And for one brief moment, I was so proud of myself."

The bonds the teens formed at a camp that treated them with dignity and respect (not to mention antibiotics) fostered self-worth and confidence the way that summer camp should. The campers grew into adults who understood that disabled people deserve the same rights and opportunities as non-disabled people. They became leaders in the disability rights movement.

When the film shows footage of Judy Heumann telling Congress, "If I have to feel thankful about an accessible bathroom, when am I ever gonna be equal in the community?" I start to get it. I didn't grow up disabled, but these are my people. Minus the gonorrhea.

Still, I maintain that there are too many advocacy days and specialty months. I'm pretty sure that even the introverts would agree that the world is better off without World Introverts Day; and furthermore, fuck Dry January. On the other hand, it occurs to me that some of these months do have merit. Black History, Women's History, Indigenous History and LGBTQIA+ Pride are initiatives that nurture confidence and dignity for their respective communities. They are the touchstones of movements that have influenced laws, legislation, attitudes and the culture. There's still work to be done, but change starts with asking for change, and asking for change means knowing your worth.

Historically speaking, people with disabilities have not been encouraged to consider their worth. It's hard not to feel cynical about the culture that has compelled us to deny or hide our disabled identities with slogans like "The Only Disability Is a Bad Attitude" and categorizations like "differently abled." Barf me to death. If we don't acknowledge that disability even exists, then we don't have to worry about how we treat disabled people.

If cultivating pride is critical to fostering a community that has the sense of worth to demand reform and the strength in numbers to make shit happen, maybe Disability Pride isn't a bullshit initiative.

Maybe embracing disability pride isn't about pretending that I enjoy having MS. (To be clear, zero stars. Do not recommend.) But hating MS is not the same as hating my body. No. Disability pride means I reject the ableist and popular notion that I should feel ashamed of my body, that I have less to contribute, that I am less able to participate in the world, that I take more than I give, that I have less inherent value and potential than the non-disabled person next to me.

In a world that insists on perfection, loving my disabled body is a radical act that promotes the idea that it's normal to be imperfect. Disability is part of who I am, and I'm proud of what I've done with these circumstances. Maybe disability pride isn't about what I've lost, or what I can't do, but a celebration of life, and a recognition that all bodies have value.

Disability pride acknowledges that I can do hard things—that I'm still here. Some days, that alone feels like enough to be proud of. It turns out there are lots of reasons to celebrate, and I realize, in fact, I *must* celebrate disability pride. Because if I can't be proud of my disabled life, then I am contributing to the idea that disability makes me less-than. That's a toxic message to put into the world—one that diminishes others with disabilities and reinforces ableist institutions. Worst of all, it's a dangerous message to give myself, and I think too highly of myself and my disabled peers to do that.

44 / I'm Not Drunk, I Have MS (Also, I'm a Little Drunk)

LATELY, IT SEEMS LIKE people assume I can't do anything for myself, and it's getting in my head. "My Uber driver just tried to buckle my seat belt," I text Tracy on my way to meet her at the salon. Four out of five trips in a stranger's vehicle inevitably include some version of disability small talk, like the classic icebreakers "what happened to your leg?" or "did you fall down?" When I'm in a good mood I let it slide, knowing the city's ride-share drivers endure their own share of micro-aggressions. They've all been asked, "so, where are you from? Like, *originally*," but this is the second time a driver has tried to buckle me in and I just want to say, *Are you fucking serious?* I text a string of eye-roll emojis to Tracy instead.

When I arrive at the nail bar, Tracy is already here, saving me my usual seat next to the nail polish display that I will use for support as I climb into the not-even-remotely-accessible pedicure chair once I've picked a colour to match the outfit I've chosen for her party. It doesn't take long to make a decision, "Hooker Red" being the only real option for a bachelorette party.

I abandon my rollator at the base of Pedicure Mountain, where a row of chairs sit four feet from the ground, like thrones. I use my arms to lift my left leg, then the right, but there's still one more step to go before I reach the summit. I repeat the process, then turn my body so that I can slide my bum onto the seat before hauling my legs up after me. The whole process takes a minute, which feels like twenty, as a salon full of yoga moms watch in rapt attention, holding their lattes and collective breath as I shimmy, limb by limb, onto the chair. When my bum finally lands safely in my seat, each and every one of those Lululemon bitches cheers like I'm a toddler taking my first steps. Tracy doesn't say a word. She doesn't have to. I know exactly what she's thinking: *Blink twice and*

I will slit the tires of their BMWs on my way out. Her psychic support is all I need to be convinced that a little humiliation merits having my toes tended to.

A day of pampering isn't what it used to be. No sufficient word exists to describe the pain of dysesthesia. My feet are medically cold. My toes barely warm up in the spa's tub of what I presume is hot water. My toenails are the colour of frostbite and the aesthetician tries to scrub off what she imagines are the remnants of blue polish (and not a sneak peek at my future corpse feet). Pedicures trigger spasticity, which causes my legs to seize, and/or clonus, an abnormal reflex that makes my feet bounce uncontrollably. I tend to tip extra if it even seems like I might kick my pedicurist in the face.

"Are you excited for your bachelorette?" I ask, trying to adjust my attitude. This day is about Tracy. Actually, this whole weekend is about Tracy. The bachelorette is still two days away. There's no way I have the energy for spa treatments and a night on the town without a rest day in between. As maid of honour, I get to set the pace, and the pace is geriatric. So in a way, I guess this weekend is also about me.

"You know I don't need a big thing," Tracy says, exasperatingly. Tracy is the opposite of a bridezilla. When it comes to wedding traditions, her approach is decidedly "whatever." I had to beg her to let me throw her a shower. The only wedding detail she insists on is that her beloved granny be at the ceremony, which means Tracy is saying her vows in the party room of Myrtle's long-term care facility.

I'm not planning anything crazy for the bachelorette anyway. In fact, I'm responsible only for the classy parts of the festivities. Champagne and selfies at my place, then cocktails at the Broadview Hotel's glass-walled rooftop bar. I left the bawdier elements of this shindig up to the other bridesmaids, the 905ers.

Which isn't to say that I'm too classy to get wild. Tracy and I have a glorious history of celebrating any number of occasions with alcohol poisoning, but we're adults now. Technically we were adults then too. We met in our twenties, but I for one can't handle the sauce like I used to. Gone are the days when I could fall down a flight of stairs on my way to the bathroom at the Snooty Fox on St. Patrick's Day, leap to my feet, throw my arms in the air and exclaim, "I'm okay!" Mary Katherine Gallagher–style.

There's no rule that says you can't drink if you have MS, but it's important to know that if you do indulge, the MS tax may apply. When drinking can temporarily compound MS symptoms, alcohol hits differently. Alcohol is a diuretic, which means alcohol makes you pee more frequently. Booze is a bladder irritant, and the baseline mood of my MS bladder is already kind of pissy. Binge-drinking Strike One.

"I'm not drunk, I have MS" is a popular saying that I didn't invent. It's ubiquitous because the sloppy gait MS causes—it attacks balance and coordination—looks a lot like the walk of a drunk. Having MS means I'm already two drinks ahead, and binge-drinking Strike Two is that alcohol can impair gait function even further.

Binge-drinking Strike Three is that drinking jacks up the fatigue that already resides deep within my old-lady bones. As for Strike Three and a Half, MS or not, literally every medical expert agrees that binge drinking is never safe or advisable. So there's that.

I'm not throwing shade at anyone who wants to toss back a glass of wine (or three). MS takes so much and each of us has to decide the pros and cons of life's pleasures. Sometimes testing our limits feels worth it.

I don't need alcohol to have a good time, but being the only sober bridesmaid at a bachelorette sucks.

IT'S CLOSE TO MIDNIGHT, which means our party has been drinking since it was still light out, back when the pre-gaming started at my apartment. While the girls chased champagne with penis-shaped Jell-O shots (courtesy of the 905ers), I took tiny sips of water out of a wine glass. I knew the night ahead would take stamina, and I refused to be the reason it might end early. I was painfully sober while we played pin the genitals on a life-sized poster of the groom, and I didn't even win that game.

We're currently the least classy table in the classy bar. The girls are hammered, and I'm having fun, but I'm also a little jealous. Tracy looks lovely in her pretty V-neck dress with the modest hemline and the cherry print. In general, Tracy's style is feminine and practical; smart, never flashy; she's not interested in being the centre of attention. Ever. Which means she's currently drunk as fuck, because it was not hard for the 905ers to talk her into a rhinestone tiara, a dollar-store sash that says "bride," and a sceptre tipped with a considerably larger-than-average pink plastic penis.

Though I am about to turn into a pumpkin, I feel proud of myself for making sure I'd last all night. The marathoning is over, I don't have to save myself for any more shenanigans. I can finally have one drink, then sleep off my exhaustion tomorrow.

I order a Manhattan—straight up, with whisky, not bourbon. It arrives in a faux-antique coupe that's full to the brim with a deep burgundy potion topped with a brandy-soaked cherry on a spear. I lean over the table, closing the gap between the drink and my mouth, unwilling to spill a single drop. I have earned this glorious drink. The first sip has the desired impact. Boozy, warm, a little bitter, hella strong. Perfection. I finish my cocktail and order another.

"To the bride!" I say, feeling overcome by thoughts of two decades of friendship. With Tracy on the cusp of a massive life change, I suddenly feel desperate to hang on to this ridiculous moment (though I refuse to touch that sceptre). I'm not afraid of how our friendship will change, I'm just experiencing a heightened awareness of how time marches on, and about the changes that are happening to me.

THE SMELL OF BLEACH is a vaguely comforting testament to the relative cleanliness of the hotel bar's bathroom floor. Meanwhile, the hum and harshness of the fluorescent lighting and the cold hard tile are sobering. Not that I need sobering, though no one would believe me. I'm not sure I believe myself. I will admit to being literally tipsy, but the haters could argue that I am, more accurately, fall-down drunk.

The Manhattans were my most recent bad decision, but my first mistake was my choice of underwear. I lost my balance trying to pull down my skin-tight slip and stumbled backwards over (and kind of into?) the waist-high garbage can. And that's how I ended up huffing bleach on the floor. All because I am incapable of putting comfort and practicality ahead of style. Well, that and also alcohol. MS was a factor, but I think we can all agree I did this to myself.

I should know better.
I do know better.
This is my fault.

I do a quick scan to make sure I'm not hurt, then decide to pick myself up. But when I try to move my legs, I can't. Panic joins shame in the group chat.

"Fuck," I say, under my breath, as I look around for something I can grab on to. The floor is littered with the contents of my wristlet—a couple of caths, a lipstick, my credit card and phone, which, like the metal grab bar that's bolted to the wall, is too far for me to reach. My rollator is close by, but it's on wheels. It's not stable, so it's useless to help me get up off the ground.

The viable option is to drag myself to the lidless, unflushed toilet and embrace it with all my might. *Gag.* What if I slip and my arm goes in the bowl? What if my face does? I label the toilet option "Plan B." My legs are so heavy that I'm not sure I could crawl anyway.

I check in with Logical Ardra, who reminds me that this is a restroom. A place to rest. I remember how when I was a kid and my Game Boy would run out of battery, I could wait five minutes, turn it back on and then get two more minutes of action. I try to do the human version of that.

I stay very still and count to sixty in my head five times over (figuring out "60 × 5" would waste precious energy). Five minutes on the floor is a long time, and I give up halfway into round three. Logical Ardra has been edged out by Impatient Ardra, who also suggests I try prayer.

"Please, please move," I beg my non-compliant legs. They still don't budge. I'm thinking about asking Siri to call 911 when someone knocks on the door.

"Occupied," I say, because *just a minute* is an unrealistic estimation.

"Ard?" It's Tracy. "Are you okay?" she asks.

By some miracle, the automatic door opener is just within my reach (though a better miracle would have been to suddenly acquire two fully functioning legs). I stretch my arm out and rally enough strength to push the big round button. The door opens excruciatingly slowly, and I half-expect sunbeams to stream in while a choir of angels sings in three-part harmony, heralding my saviour's arrival. Instead, I hear the muted bass of the nightclub down the hall. Tracy is alone. *Hallelujah, she didn't bring the 905ers.*

"I'm so sorry, Trace. This is your night and I'm the messy one. I shouldn't have had that second drink. Or the first one."

"Shut up. I'm glad you had fun." Tracy reads the situation. She collects my stuff from the floor. "You want me to throw this out?" she asks about the lipstick, since the lid came off. I nod, while Tracy looks at me appraisingly. "Hold this," she says, handing me the penis sceptre. Gross, but I don't protest. Her body language screams *I'm in charge now*. Tracy moves behind me and slips her hands under my armpits. On the count of three she pulls me into a standing position in one smooth motion with what seems like a refined technique, like she's been training for this moment.

"Thank you for rescuing me. I feel like such an idiot."

"Jesus, stop gushing. It's part of the job."

"Of being my best friend?"

"You would do the same for me."

"We would both end up on the floor."

"You know what I mean!" Tracy laughs. I do. "Let's get you in an Uber," she says, then texts The Banker, telling him I'm on my way and to meet me at the door of our building. When my car arrives, she puts my rollator in the trunk, then taps me on the forehead with the penis sceptre like some deviant fairy godmother. "Thank you for an awesome night!" she says, without any attempt to buckle my seat belt.

45 / At Least It's Not Cancer

DARCY AND I ARE OPTIMISTS. We count our blessings, kiss our dogs, we believe in love. We both agree that life is worth living. At least for now. We're also realists. MS isn't getting easier, and neither Darcy nor I make any promises that we'll be able to exist in our decomposing bodies indefinitely. We assume MS will drive us to our thresholds eventually. And then what?

"Hope you get cancer!" Darcy trills.

"I hope *you* get cancer!" I whisper back before hanging up. The Banker is within earshot, and I don't want to have to answer any WTF-was-that-all-about questions. The tongue-in-cheek sign-off we've recently adopted is only partly inspired by the ever-pervasive idea that if you happen to have MS you should be grateful that "at least it's not cancer." Like it's one or the other instead of neither, or both.

Never mind that not all cancer is the same, just as not all MS is the same. Or that some MS treatments can actually make you more susceptible to cancer. "At least it's not cancer" is a tired refrain people repeat when they don't know what else to say. Or maybe they just want you to shut up and stop complaining. The darker truth behind the (un)well wishes Darcy and I exchange isn't really about how much we'd like to throat-punch the "at least" people anyway, if only we had the strength.

Although it's true some cancer can make you die, MS is off the hook for being labelled terminal, because most people stop living from "causes related to MS" as opposed to MS itself—a technicality some people find comforting—but I think dead is dead. Statistically, MS shaves roughly eight years off of life expectancy, which sounds a lot to me like MS is, in fact, coming for you, albeit eventually. MS-adjacent deaths are caused by things like choking, sepsis, aspirational pneumonia or falling down six flights of stairs.

Usually, the eight-year advance discharge is delivered like it's good news, with a heavy emphasis on the word *only*. Like we're not supposed to care about the crappy years at the end. But eight years is the lifespan of the average Saint Bernard, and I for one am not comforted by the thought of MS shortening my life by one whole dog.

Meanwhile, MS is marketed as a manageable condition. Ever since higher-efficacy medications have come on the scene, life expectancies are increasing. It's true that some people are living with MS well into old age. One of my favourite *Tripping on Air* stans is octogenarian Edie, who's had MS for roughly seven hundred years. But we never hear about the presumably unpleasant late-stage years of those with advanced symptoms. In addition to life-enders like sepsis and his murdering side-kicks, frailty and asphyxiation, the risk of suicide in the MS population is twice that of the general public. The truth that no one talks about is that for some people, MS can become so severely disabling that life becomes unbearable.

My MS and Darcy's are on separate trajectories, of course, but neither of us has been among the lucky whose disease has been relatively quiet. Still, on our best days, we leave room for the possibility of improvements, of long-term stability. We have learned to adapt and not die. Darcy especially believes—way more than I do—that a cure is on the horizon, but I don't think it's unreasonable to dip a mostly numb toe into the water of Worst-Case What-Ifs from time to time.

Should symptoms become too much for either of us to handle, Darcy and I agree that suicide is too horrifying to merit true consideration. Death by out-of-control cancer, on the other hand, seems like a convenient end to any potential insufferable suffering. Succumbing to an imaginary illness with a heaping side of morphine is a shared fantasy for Darcy and me, because managing MS indefinitely feels more far-fetched to us than surviving it, and I will probably delete this chapter because my mother, at least, is going to freak out that I am trying to manifest cancer.

My mom can relax. For one thing, Darcy and I are not witches. Furthermore, we don't have a suicide pact. We're not taking up smoking, or playing with X-ray machines; we're not shopping the dark web for boxes of asbestos. Nobody's actively pursuing cancer. Even if I am ignoring an aberrant mole on my face—I'm still wearing sunscreen! Thinking about my mortality is not the same as giving all my stuff away and drafting a breakup letter to life. The occasional existential inventory helps me get on with it. No need to call any hotlines.

Medical assistance in dying (MAID) has been legal in Canada since 2016, but it's not until 2021, when a "reasonably foreseeable death" ceases to be an eligibility requirement, that Darcy and I start to pay attention. MS is added to the list of qualifying conditions, and though it feels like a weird thing to get excited about, here we are.

I'm not looking to check out anytime soon, but knowing that someday I *could* grants me a feeling of, I don't know, relief? Until MAID became available for people like me, my end-of-life plan involved a last-ditch trip to Switzerland, the no-questions-asked assisted suicide capital of the world, where the appeal of death by drug-laced chocolate is tempered by the cruelty of dying with jet lag.

("Really? They do it with chocolate?" TB interrupts when I read him this chapter. OMG, obviously not. You have to pay extra for that.)

Now that a self-determined death is just a bit of paperwork and a phone call away, Switzerland is off the table and I can trade my Air Miles for Amazon gift cards. Darcy and I can start using our wishes for practical things, like wishing for more wishes.

But before we pop the champagne on Canada's landmark ruling, a tiny part of my brain wonders if I'm actually okay with being on a federally sanctioned list of Reasons to Die. It's one thing for me to panic and catastrophize about what MS might do to me; I say all kinds of crazy shit.

When the government says, "Yeah, we don't think you should have to live like this; in fact, we're gonna change the law so that you won't have to," it's as validating as it is unnerving. If the words *you can do this* are sometimes enough to make me believe that I can, in fact, keep going, isn't it possible that the words *you don't have to* could have just as much of an impact?

These are heavy contemplations. A problem for Future Me. MAID still feels far away and theoretical, like my retirement savings or clean hair day. We're all going to die, but none of us actually believes it. I mean, not really. I put my eventual demise out of my mind until a full year later, when I hear from Jenny, a reader of *Tripping on Air*.

Jenny looks like a California blonde, though she is Canadian. Tall and lean, her body appears to have been built by yoga and lemon water. A former athlete, equestrienne and artist, Jenny no longer has the hand and arm strength to paint. Jenny is a self-described tough bitch, but lately she feels like her MS symptoms rule her day and have stripped her of her sense of purpose.

Jenny offers me a physiotherapy device that's no longer helping her. I accept because I love free stuff, but giving your shit away is right up there with clearing your browser history as a classic sign of preparing to jump ship. It's the reason I don't trust Marie Kondo.

Sure enough, Jenny tells me in a follow-up email that she's applied for MAID.

Jenny sends me her physio device with a series of instructional videos she's filmed. I start to doubt that the device will help when I see how much better Jenny's mobility is than my own. Her dorsiflexion is enviable. I'm filled with confusion as I watch her foot lift to a forty-five-degree angle. Jenny doesn't use her arms to move her legs, like I do. Jenny stands without a mobility aid and walks across the *carpeted floor.* (Carpeted!) I know that Jenny often uses a scooter to get around and I don't doubt that Jenny's MS symptoms are fucking up her life, but she is not the picture of pre-dead I expected. Despite what I know about invisible illness, I can't help but wonder how the eff Jenny could be approved for MAID.

"Grievous suffering" is subjective. I remember how enraged I felt when Dr. Muppet assessed me as "not as bad as you think you are." The math on how much you are suffering is precisely the amount you *believe* yourself to be suffering. It's not up to me (thank God) to decide what is or isn't tolerable for someone else. Jenny doesn't owe me her reasons, never mind her definition of what's reasonable, but she agrees to let me interview her for the blog.

Over a lengthy Zoom call, Jenny assures me she does not have depression. I ask if she would feel less fatalistic if she had access to better home care, work opportunities, accessible spaces—if there was less stigma around chronic illness. She looks back at me blankly, like she hasn't considered these things, because they're so obviously out of reach. I ask what it would mean if the doctor who had left her undiagnosed for ten treatable years were to apologize, and she wells up. I have to wonder if the system that is willing to help Jenny die has done enough to help her live.

On the opposite side of the mood board, Jenny's approval for MAID coincides with a chance for her to have HSCT. She knows how risky the procedure is—the stakes are life or death—but she feels she has nothing to lose. HSCT has been used in clinical trials in Canada since 2000, but by 2022, it's still not available to patients like Jenny (or Darcy, or Sherry, or my cousin Kyle, or my friend Carrie, or my brother-in-law Shawn, or me). Jenny must travel to Mexico on the considerable dime of her friends.

Jenny has no beef with MAID, but others do: there's blowback from the online chronic-illness community about Canada's application of the new legislation. The controversy is jarring, because it's the disabled population that MAID is supposed to benefit.

In December 2022, the CBC reports that retired corporal and Paralympian Christine Gauthier was offered an unsolicited medically assisted death (complete with the necessary equipment) by Veterans Affairs Canada in lieu of the home wheelchair ramp she'd been requesting for five years. Gauthier is not the only veteran to whom this long-term "solution" has been proposed, and stories of coercion abound. I know first-hand how often people make false assumptions about the quality of life of people with disabilities, and it's chilling to think about who exactly is doling out life-ending advice.

I am well acquainted with the patience required to be a patient in this country. I've been on a physiotherapy wait-list for almost two years now. I stress about the impact of insufficient PT on my degree of disability. It's upsetting to realize that while I continue to wait for a spot to open up in rehab, I could be approved for MAID in just ninety days.

In addition to complaints of insufficient, under-resourced health care, a staggering number of disabled people point out the critical lack of adequate accessible housing that is driving them to seek out MAID. With so many sick people struggling to simply exist on a disability income that keeps them in poverty, it's hard to believe that policy-makers are ultimately concerned with "dignity." When death is the alternative to a properly funded health-care system, it starts to feel kinda eugenics-y.

I am rattled into renewed appreciation for my relative privilege. TB's insurance covers ninety-five per cent of the $940.38 a month my catheters cost (that's $4.47 per pee). We have a mostly accessible place to live. I can afford uberASSIST and don't have to rely on Wheel-Trans if I have to get across town on my own. "Can you believe this thing costs three-hundred dollars?" is how I introduce my pressure-sore pillow to everyone who encounters it. It's not a flex, it's just a mind-boggling amount to spend on a cushion, and I feel the need to say it out loud every chance I get. I resent how much of our disposable income goes to funding my sick-girl lifestyle, but I know that I am lucky enough that when I need a little treat to get me through a difficult Patient Day, we don't have to miss any meals or dip into our overdraft to be able to afford it.

Which isn't to say we're living completely fancy-free. Well, at least one of us isn't. I don't think of my retirement savings because I believe in "seize the day" and "it's just money, you can get more," but The Banker has a different perspective. He doesn't say anything about how much I spend on essentials like Starbucks and manicures, but when it's time to do our taxes, he argues the pros and cons of squirrelling any surplus into an investment vehicle (to him, there are no cons), while I argue for something more immediately essential, like a vacation, or a new hat.

I'm not sure what I'll need beyond prescription meds, mobility aids, medical supplies and help around the house once TB retires and his insurance expires. I don't want to think about the potential need for Hoyer Lifts or personal care workers, so I don't. My plan to cover the cost of catheters is to just pee less. Which is why I'm getting my drinking in now. Like a camel.

I don't want my husband to, at some point, have to turn into my nurse. I always thought we would outsource any help I might need, but in researching the top reasons people choose MAID, I'm learning that home-care costs can quickly rack up to hundreds of dollars a day. Darcy had a recent fall that set her back considerably. Now she's fighting the system to secure enough home care to keep her out of a long-term care facility where she would be the youngest resident by decades.

That MS might shorten my life by one whole dog feels tragic, but beyond my control. The idea that anyone might not be able to afford to live with MS is actually sickening. Just thinking about it makes me want to bury my anxiety in a new sweater, an extravagance I justify, because what's the difference? How many sweaters would I need to not buy to be able to finance a so-called life of dignity?

Fortunately, Jenny's stem cell transplant is a success, and being approved for medical assistance in dying doesn't mean you're obligated to follow through. The Grim Reaper doesn't show up at your door with a pre-filled syringe and a body bag. But MAID doesn't have a lot of guardrails either. Jenny still has MS, and though her circumstances have fundamentally changed, her approval for MAID is valid for ten years without considering the reason why hotel windows don't open and bridges have barriers.

Jenny is the first person with MS in my orbit to have pursued MAID, but she won't be the last. MAID is supposed to be a last resort, but Jenny wasn't offered any other options. It was up to her to figure out and finance HSCT on her own. Unlike doctors in Belgium and the Netherlands, where MAID is also available, Canadian doctors are not required to have exhausted all treatment alternatives before approving patients for MAID. In a world where suicide is considered the pinnacle of irrationality, and disability is considered a fate worse than death, we aren't doing nearly enough to make the lives of the disabled more livable.

My enthusiasm for MAID was naive. I assumed that a medically assisted death was merely an alternative to unimaginable physical suffering, not a means to end suffering caused by social inequities.

Darcy and I no longer need to whisper our secret death wishes. MAID has quickly become so normalized that my concern about being overheard now has more to do with whichever random bureaucrat might agree my life isn't worth living. I'm not anti-MAID, but the program, and our culture in general, could use a bit more scrutiny. I still may use MAID someday, but in the meantime, it seems like my energy would be better spent advocating for change and figuring out how to mitigate the modifiable factors that put me at a higher risk for wanting off this planet.

I don't know what my threshold will be, but for now I recognize that even on my worst days, a snuggle with the dog, a phone call with a friend, my husband's hand on my leg while we watch TV are comforts that make life feel worth living. I can't just roll the dice on the things I can control. I have a responsibility to look after myself. The next time I talk to Darcy I tell her about the sketchy mole on my face. "Ard," she says, dead serious, "you really should get that checked out. You don't want cancer."

I agree.

46 / Mourning Routine

GOOD MORNING? I don't know how to start the day in a good—or at least not hostile—mood when from the literal moment I wake up I have problems to solve, and the problems are me.

Getting out of bed doesn't just happen, it's a multi-step process. There's no "up and at 'em." First, I grab my pyjama pants and a handful of thigh to pull my left leg up, hoping the movement won't cause my right leg to seize. Still on my back, once both legs are bent at the knee, I un-Velcro the calf-high boots that keep my ankles from inverting in the night, then toss the boots on the floor. The tear of Velcro is the first sound I hear in the morning and the last sound I hear at night. I shimmy into a sitting position and try not to slide off the bed. Most of the time I make it.

The Banker, who has been up for who knows how long before me, understands it's time to start the coffee when he hears the slow clomp of two canes on the hardwood as I make my way to the bathroom. My clothes are already there—a recent life hack that saves me some steps. I keep my socks and underwear in baskets under the sink. Some women get dressed in fancy walk-in closets. I get dressed on the toilet because it's low to the ground and less difficult for me to lift my legs into pants.

It takes twenty minutes to change from nighttime pyjamas to their daytime equivalent: track pants and the T-shirt I will later sleep in (yet another life hack). I blast my hair with dry shampoo and marvel at how much energy it takes to look like I haven't made an effort at all. If my socks go on upside down, so that the little extra fabric for the heel is uncomfortably on the top of my ankle, so be it. My legs are spent, heavy and useless; my arms are tired; and my will is too weak to lift my ankle up onto my knee again. I start the day already defeated. By a fucking sock.

Next up, the stress-fest of breakfast. I enter the kitchen knowing that on any given day there's a good chance I will drop X, spill Y, forget Z. It's been months since I've had one of the nutrient-dense smoothies that were once a staple of my routine. I could have cereal, but the bananas are inconveniently located on the counter opposite the bowls, which seems like an easy enough problem to solve, but the kettle is screaming. It's full, and I won't be able to lift it. I've been burned before. I slide the kettle off of the stove and leave The Banker to deal with it. I try to get myself some orange juice but my hand isn't strong enough to open the plastic lip on the container.

When TB says, "Good morning," I have to decide which version of me he's gonna get: frustrated, angry or artificially cheerful. I've never been a morning person, but when every day starts with a struggle, how can that not inform my mood?

It's been roughly thirteen years since we made Toronto our home. Thirteen years of hosting parties, playing cards on the balcony, bingeing our favourite shows with the dog snuggled up next to us on the overstuffed couch. I love this city, our neighbourhood, our home. Also, I want out.

Maybe I could have predicted that the nine-foot library ladder would someday become a hazard, but I am caught off guard by all the ways our home begins to disable me. The once-luxurious soaker tub now feels like a potential coffin when I can't climb in and out of it. The shower isn't a great alternative. There's a lip to get in and I lose my balance whenever I close my eyes. I cut my hand on the sharp end of a towel rack after using it as a grab bar. *Should I be worried about tetanus?*

It's no longer possible to get up on a chair to reach something from a high cupboard, though we still keep a chair in the kitchen in case I need to take a break while getting a snack. I don't have my coffee on the balcony anymore if I'm alone. For one thing, it's hard to carry a beverage when you're using two canes to walk, and clearing the half-step up to the outdoor space requires me to have a spotter.

As for the neighbourhood, the location is great, but what does it matter when I haven't left the house in a week?

The Banker and I hack what we can. One by one, he gets rid of the carefully curated housewares that have come to feel like weapons of self-destruction. Drop foot makes me trip on everything, so the area rugs and even the front door mat have to go. He adds sliding drawers to cupboards and an industrial-strength magnet to hold open the heavy front door so that I can keep my hands on my rollator while exiting and entering the apartment. I order a stepstool to keep next to the bed. A shower bench and a handlebar help me in and out of the tub. The bathroom counter really doesn't have room for a hair-dryer stand, but I get one anyway.

I resent all of my disability decor. The tools I need to navigate the space are not pleasing to look at. They certainly don't spark joy and I would pay double for this stuff if the manufacturers made any of it look less medical. Worse than my resentment, though, is the anger that shows up when I'm feeling especially sidelined by my home—the place where I'm supposed to feel the safest. When I fail to do something simple like open the lid to the fucking orange juice, it makes me want to break something. I want to hurl the juice at the wall. If only I had the strength.

I consult two contractors to see if we can renovate the bathroom. The biggest threat to my safety, energy and hygiene is our inaccessible ensuite. I figure that my most urgent problem would be solved if we could take out the tub and build a roll-in shower. The first contractor I speak with sighs when he sees the space. He tells me we'd have to rip out a wall, devalue the property. There's not much room to work with and he doesn't want to do it. The second guy is more thoughtful. I tell him I'm looking for long-term solutions so that I can stay in the home that I love. He gently asks me why I would go to the expense of making the bathroom accessible when the narrow kitchen, with its high cupboards and lack of turning radius, isn't accessible at all.

TB and I start looking at other units in our building, but they all have the same problems. We search for real estate in our neighbourhood, but the availability of truly accessible housing is almost non-existent.

Hope is renewed when I learn that Toronto has an accessible housing real estate expert. He even wrote a book! *Barrier Free Real Estate: Achieving Freedom at Home* by Jeffrey Kerr. One of Jeff's top tips is to find an apartment or condo with a gym in the building because a gym will have accessible bathrooms. My head wants to explode. It's not Jeff's fault that accessible housing is so scarce that "just shower in the gym" is a good enough idea that it deserves to be in a book. Surely we can do better than this.

There's a new building under construction and it's just around the corner from our current apartment. TB and I decide to start from scratch. We enlist the help of Jeff and head to the sales office where we meet Helena, a senior design consultant who works for the developer. When Helena sees my mobility aid, she's keen to tell me that new builds are required to make 15 percent of units barrier-free. New buildings must be designed to be accessible and adaptable! This means including features like wider doorways, lower light switches, roll-in showers, and reinforced walls that can support the installation of grab bars and lifts. I'm excited enough that I let it slide when she uses terms like *wheelchair bound* and *confinement* even though I think someone tasked with describing accessibility features should have a better handle on the language of disability.

Mandating accessibility feels pretty cool and progressive until I stop to think about the fact that 15 percent is actually kinda low, considering the scarcity of barrier-free housing combined with the fact that the disabled and aging populations far exceed 15 percent. What's worse, Helena tells us that barrier-free units get scooped up quickly. They're especially popular because of their enormous bathrooms, and anyone can buy them. It blows my mind that there's no obligation for developers to ensure that the units are allocated to people who really need them. It's like having accessible parking that anyone can use.

Nonetheless, hope's not dead yet. We consider a smattering of floorplans and find a small two-bedroom, two-bathroom unit that's within our budget. But the design is confusing.

"The ensuite looks tiny," I say. "How is this accessible?"

"Oh," Helena says, "we're only required to make *part* of the unit accessible."

"So, the main bedroom and bathroom aren't designed to be barrier-free? They have narrow doors and no turning radius?"

"The walls aren't reinforced either."

It's so insulting. As if anyone who chooses to live in an eight-hundred-square-foot apartment wouldn't want the option of entering the whole space, let alone the main bedroom and bathroom.

I refuse to live in some partially accessible, modern-day Bluebeard's castle, where certain rooms are off-limits to me, so we put a deposit on the new build and assume the added cost of making the whole apartment accessible. I know how lucky I am to be able to do this. Canada, like so many other countries, has a serious housing crisis and Toronto in particular suffers from a lack of acceptable options.

Now we wait a few years for construction to finish, crossing our fingers that my health remains relatively stable and that our new home is ready before I fall in the tub or trip on the balcony, or simply become more disabled and our current place becomes unsustainable.

47 / Independence Day

IT'S EARLY SPRING, so basically the throes of winter in Toronto. The Banker and I are overdue for a break—not from each other—but from work, the city, the grind. The break I really need is from MS, but MS doesn't stop for coffee, let alone a vacation. The message MS leaves on my voice mail: *Ooh, sorry, I'm saving up for a conflict diamond and a coat made of puppy fur, so I'm actually working overtime. I'm on my way downtown right now to see if we can't squeeze in another UTI! See you at 3 a.m. for your nerve-pain appointment! TTFN.*

Wherever I go, MS is coming with me, but I figure staring at a lake and a fireplace with a bowl of Merlot in hand and a dog in my lap might take some of the edge off. Northern Ontario is full of cozy high-end cottages, but you need to book them seven years in advance and I failed to predict my burnout, so we're headed to the only last-minute option, a "boutique motel," instead.

When we arrive, the gravel parking lot is covered with ice that has melted and refrozen. The walkway that's kind of shovelled, but mostly not, isn't wide enough for my rollator. I navigate slippery, uneven terrain to get to our "accessible" room, while my unpaid porter (The Banker) unloads my considerable baggage from the car. I already feel pissy and unwelcome but these are not vacation vibes. I try to keep my attitude in check.

While the dog sniffs out the place like she's gunning for a job at the airport, I take in the room from my position, flopped out on the bed. The bathroom is tiny enough that I will have to leave my mobility aid outside the door. There's no fireplace, no lake view, no hot tub (or any tub). There's no lounging in two-hundred-dollar robes on down-filled duvets while gazing at mountains or a sunset over a lake. This is a crash pad for people who enjoy cold exercise and have two fully functioning legs. I've brought us to a town for skiers, and we're not here to ski. We're not even here to have sex. I've been coping with unrelenting GI pain for weeks and have no energy to do anything remotely active. I feel like an asshole for insisting we spend money just to lie around and look at four different walls and a TV that's smaller than the one we have at home. "Boutique motel" doesn't mean luxury, and I blame *Schitt's Creek* for the confusion.

The Banker does the work of getting us settled while I try to calculate how long I should wait before asking him to move the area rugs that threaten to trip me. I could use a glass of water, but I'm still figuring out if my thirst is greater than my desire to not be annoying. Mentally triaging my wants versus needs before half asking, half apologizing for small favours has become part of my personality lately. *Since you're up, could I trouble you to adjust the pillow under my feet? Babe, would you mind plugging in the heating blanket, covering my right foot (but not the left), throwing out this handful of used Kleenex and turning up the heat?*

"Can you help me take my pants off in a non-sexy way?" is a real thing that I have asked.

I might sound like a pampered princess with a manservant in my employ, but more often than not, these words taste like bile in my mouth. Asking for help every time I get trapped in my sweater or can't get up off the floor is demoralizing. But again, we are not here so that I can feel sorry for myself. We are here to watch a tiny TV and eat takeout in bed, because these are not our sheets and we do not have to clean them.

Normally my husband and I argue over pickup versus delivery. TB hates to spend money on extra fees, but I would pay double for the most minor convenience. Google Maps tells us the sole takeout option is literally a two-minute drive away, so in this case I don't put up a fight. TB will pick up our order. He'll be back in a jiffy.

Forty-five minutes later, I start to wonder what the actual fuck is a jiffy. I reach for my phone to learn some etymology before remembering that it's charging on the other side of the bed. Since sliding and scooching are no longer movements my body consents to, I would have to get my rollator to make the journey to my phone. No thanks. I decide a jiffy is however long TB's been gone plus five more minutes, then watch the digital clock for three minutes before I let myself start to freak out.

Reasonable Me knows that I am about to get pretty unreasonable. The Banker is slow, he lives in his own decelerated time zone and talks to absolutely everyone. He should see a doctor about his dyschronometria. He also sucks at directions, even with GPS. In all likelihood, TB has accidentally taken the scenic route or is chatting with the restaurant staff. I could confirm this if I were willing to get up and text "u alive," but I'm in the mood to fuck myself up. I decide to instead play What's the Worst That Could Happen?

Maybe The Banker got hit by a falling icicle in the parking lot. What if a bear, emerging from hibernation, attacked him for his takeout? Did he pick up a hitchhiker, only to realize they have a lot in common, and now they're best friends on a cross-country road trip?

I can't believe TB would desert me, which means he's obviously dead. I imagine the phone call: *Ma'am, we found a man lying in a parking lot in a pool of water. We've got a bear here, says he's allergic to peanuts and couldn't have attacked anyone for their pad Thai. Also, a guy with a stick and bag tied to the end of it. Name's Hobo Hank. Says he's next of kin.*

I'm spiralling. Bears probably don't even like pad Thai, but fifteen people in America are killed by falling icicles each year. Unfortunately, I don't have time to dwell on funeral arrangements. I have to figure out how to fend for myself.

There are two granola bars in my bag, so starvation, at least, isn't imminent. I don't drive. I'm not strong enough to put our luggage in the car. I'm not even strong enough to walk the dog, who's reading this situation and staring out the window, trying to manifest The Banker's return. There's no way this hick town has Uber. Even if they have Uber Tractor or Uber Snowmobile, how will I get back to Toronto? (Later, Tracy interrupts this part of my story to say, "Obviously, I would have picked you up," because a true best friend legitimizes your semi-psychotic breakdowns.)

Three hours from home, trapped in a motel, *Misery*-style, MS is my Annie Wilkes. I feel incapable. I feel like a child, and not even the child version of myself, because I was a pretty self-sufficient kid—like one of those Japanese kindergarteners who takes the subway and does the family's taxes.

I force myself to think of Darcy, my touchstone in an MS crisis. Even after she became a full-time powerchair user, Darcy figured out how to live on her own. She CEOs the shit out of her life, managing her care like a boss. She even has a dog. Granted, it's a little dog, but it's not like she had to settle for a cat.

If TB has indeed moved on to the afterlife, I know that people would help me. Just different people from the person who's already been helping the most. And that is the root of my freakout. I don't know when the scale tipped exactly, when living independently became unrealistic. I haven't bothered to tease apart courtesies and small favours from the tasks I am truly incapable of doing on my own. When my husband says, "Let me pour you a glass of wine," it doesn't have the same effect on me as "Let me clean the bathroom (because if I don't, no one will)."

TB lets me believe he's peeling grapes and making me HWBs (hot water bottles) because he's chivalrous, romantic, decent. He doesn't labour like he's staff or give himself props for keeping me alive. But I can't remember the last time I did the laundry or the dishes. I tell myself I'm independent without considering that there's no way I could scrub the floors, clean the tub, take out the garbage. Even when I order food, if TB isn't home, I struggle to get the delivery off the doorstep and into the apartment.

I freely acknowledge my dependence on Netflix and Amazon. I'm not ashamed to admit that I once DoorDash'd an Americano from Starbucks. (Okay, it was more than once, and I am a little ashamed.) But when I think about my dependence on another person to pick up my Amazon packages and to get the Miss Vickies chips off the high shelf, my chest tightens. I feel powerless being at the mercy of someone else.

TB is (probably) fine. My panic, though, is not completely unfounded. The truth my motel epiphany reveals is that in an actual emergency, I would be limited by what I could do.

"Sorry that took so long. They don't check online orders, so nothing was ready when I got there," TB says as he enters the room, alive and with an armful of food, oblivious to the multiple catastrophes he's just dodged.

"No worries," I say, without revealing my garbage bag full of concerns. I know I'm lucky to have help, but I don't feel lucky like someone who won the lottery. *Lucky* feels like a slur. I haven't yet figured out that independence isn't, in fact, a virtue, which makes confronting the reality of my neediness more painful than it needs to be.

There's more to consider than my enormous ego when figuring out how I feel about requiring help. Being disabled forces me to be vulnerable, to live with a degree of defencelessness, and to have faith that others will have my best interest at heart. Accepting help is not a choice, it's a survival skill—one that I haven't mastered yet.

48 / The C-Word

IT'S MARTINI MONDAY. The Banker and I are catching each other up on our respective workdays. He's droning on about a conversation he had with one of his banking bros and I am feigning attention. Bank talk is boring, and I'm only ever half-tuned in to office anecdotes that are devoid of any actual drama. Even with a healthier-than-average appreciation for grammar, I have zero interest in the mailer Bryan sent out that had six typos. Unless Bryan's banging the new guy or is being criminally investigated for insider trading, clerical fuck-ups are not gossip. Hard pass.

On this night, though, TB's work story starts to involve me, and that's when I perk up, "me" being my favourite subject. That is until I hear him say the word that forces me to interrupt. "I'm sorry, you told your colleague you're my *caregiver*?"

The C-word is not something I have ever heard TB say. At least not as it pertains to me. It's a good thing I have a bit of a buzz on, because I am not impressed. Not impressed at all.

Our marriage is sustained by a list of words and phrases I never want to hear. It includes intrusive questions like "How did you sleep?" (I didn't), "What time do you want to get up?" (I do not get up at "times") and "Do you want me to pick up some Miss Vickies while I'm at the store?" (duh). The list doesn't include the C-word for the same reason it doesn't include the word *moist* or the question "Wanna watch the game?" Some things go without saying. Or so I thought.

The C-word sucks, and here's some evidence to back up my thesis: According to at least one dictionary (*Merriam-Webster*), a caregiver is "a person who provides direct care (as for children, elderly people, or the chronically ill)." Okay, that's reasonable, I guess. Except that *Merriam-Webster* goes on to suggest that "the care of a patient . . . can be a physical, emotional and financial drain on the family caregiver." *Merriam-Webster* says that needing a C-word makes you a B-word: burden. *Rude.* I miss the days when I could just be a bitch and a cunt.

With the right lawyer, The Banker might actually be able to claim the moniker *caregiver*. I do have a chronic illness, and I guess "direct care" could include things like picking me up at the spa, mixing cocktails and, sure, helping me into my foot braces at night. But caring exists on a spectrum, especially when it comes to a disease as variable as MS. I don't want to diminish how much TB cares for me, but what percentage of my care is enough to qualify him as a capital-*C* Caregiver? Because, when it comes to managing my MS, it takes a village of medical professionals and social supports, and although I appreciate that TB puts the rollator in the trunk of the car 100 percent of the time (except for the two times he left it in a parking lot), I feed and dress myself, manage my appointments and make all my own medical decisions. I make all my own life decisions, and a lot of the household decisions too. Yes, he does a lot for me, but the person who is responsible for the overwhelming majority of my MS care is *me*.

Am I overreacting? Sure. You know my brand. Rejecting the label of caregiver doesn't mean a rejection of care, only that using the C-word would define our relationship by MS, and make MS the Most Important Thing. When one person's the C-word, the balance of caring is placed entirely on one side of the relationship. The C-word reinforces a parent–child dynamic and suggests I'm a dependent, incapable of providing care myself. And sure, a rose by any other name is still going to drive me to my doctors' appointments and pick up my prescriptions, but words matter, and the language we use impacts how we feel. I concede that there may come a tipping point when, someday, I need considerably more care. Using the C-word before we're even close to that point feels like a rush toward a dynamic neither of us wants.

Before I finish my drink, The Banker backs up his claim to martyrdom by giving me the full context of his foul language. "I was just explaining that I need to keep working from home for now because I'm the caregiver of someone who is at high risk for COVID and other infections," he says. Though this time around, he says the word *caregiver* much quieter. Like he's scared.

"Okay," I say, concealing my relief, "but you could have just said my *wife* is high risk." I don't bother adding that parents, partners and friends are already relationships that include an element of caring, of keeping safe. It's his first offence, and it's worth considering that *caregiver* and *high risk* are words we've been hearing repeatedly over the past couple of pandemic years.

"Yeah, that makes sense," he concedes. TB knows that my lawyer is a better lawyer than his lawyer. (My lawyer is me.)

With the C-word officially added to the Household List of Forbidden Words, I buy myself a little more time to adjust to my evolving need for care. I feel best about the role MS plays in our marriage when I think of us handling it as we would any crisis: as a team. Resisting the C-word is my way of insisting that I'm still in the game. TB might be my MVP, but I'm still the captain.

49 / I'm Ardra Shephard

"I'M ARDRA SHEPHARD and this is *Fashion Dis*, the world's first makeover series dedicated to elevating and celebrating the style and beauty potential of people with disabilities." I state it proudly, staring directly into the lens of the camera.

"Looks good, let's just do one more take for safety," the director says. I've been saying "I'm Ardra Shephard" all morning, and I'm happy to say it a hundred times more. It feels pretty fucking great to be me right now.

It's Monday, like a real, working-person Monday, assuming real people get picked up at the crack of 9:30 and chauffeured to work where someone else is tasked with brushing their hair. I am in an unrecognizably cheerful mood. I swear the sky is a different, even better kind of blue. Today is "Ardra Day" on set, which means I'm the only "talent" called. We're filming the opening, the throws, some promos and content for a sizzle reel. Saying I'm the only talent in a room of twenty or so people makes it sound like I'm a bit of an asshole who thinks PAs or grips are talentless hacks, but these aren't my words, this is industry lingo—and to be fair, I am not yet fluent. I don't even know what a grip is or does, though I assume they are human beings who hold things.

If you're wondering how the eff I ended up with a TV show, good question! That dude who emailed me after he saw my *xoJane* article? Turns out he was legit. His name is Andrew Morris and he's the director of production at Accessible Media Inc., or AMI-tv. He hired me to do some consulting on a couple of series projects for the network. I started pitching my own ideas, and now a show I created—*Fashion Dis*—is hitting the ground running. Or limping, wheeling, slow-walking. Whatever the actual speed—let's be real, nobody's running—it does feel like we're moving quickly after a couple of slow-motion years in development, when the show's working title was *Beauty for Every Body*.

It's been about a month since the pre-production meeting where I met many of the people working on the show, from the director to the

DP (whatever that means), to the on-camera style team. As each cast and crew member introduced themselves, they talked about their own connection to disability and expressed how excited they were about working on this show and realizing this vision. My vision! An idea that once lived in my heart and head has suddenly become something so much bigger than me. The experience so far has been David After Dentist–level surreal. Like, is this real life? Am I actually at the centre of a groundbreaking new show, or am I riding high on nitrous oxide?

Cara, the showrunner (industry jargon for "person who runs the show"), has the heavy blunt-cut bangs of my dreams. Her fringe is as commanding as her personality. She told the meeting that one of the perks of working on *Fashion Dis* is the more relaxed pace, because working with the disability community requires flexibility and humane work hours. Cara made it clear that this production is exceptional, though anyone who works in the industry already knows that when a show is in production, you're not seeing your kid's baseball games or taking any personal days. You'd better hope no one you love dies. It's not lost on me that non-disabled bodies also have plenty of needs, but those needs are expected to be ignored once filming has begun.

There are many barriers to the entertainment industry for people with disabilities. One of them is that a seven- or eight-hour workday is considered an accommodation. The world of television and film is notoriously workist. I'm initially impressed by perks like having a driver and all my meals provided, but it eventually occurs to me that this is an industry-wide standard that ensures the talent doesn't waste time making lunch, or going outside. The hours on a standard set are long and self-important. Ten-hour days can feel like a gift when the law says twelve hours is acceptable, as if a film set is as indispensable as a hospital. Mother Teresa can rest in peace knowing that Doctors Who, Phil and Pimple Popper are consistently putting in overtime.

I get it. I really do believe that storytelling is as essential as air and water. I'll be the first to acknowledge that changing the culture has the potential to improve and even save lives. A show that normalizes disability in the fashion and beauty space is long overdue and existentially important, but I don't think we need to keep actual physicians' hours. Of course, it's not up to me to reform the industry. I'm not sure anyone can. Except, on this show, I actually do have a voice, plus the support of the broadcast network.

The production company entrusted with making the show is Nikki Ray Media, where there's enthusiasm but no real experience working with the disability community. While we were in development I had a considerable role educating the team on what a barrier-free production would require in order to be successful. A Disability Screen Office is a much-needed industry resource that, in 2021, is still a couple of years away from existing. The beach-day vibes Cara promised at the production meeting are a six- to eight-hour marathon for me (and still a ten- to twelve-hour day for the crew). This might be a slower pace by industry standards, but I've been medically retired since 2005. I've spent the past nine months trying to establish a reliable-ish bowel routine just so that I can get out the door at 9:30.

Although I'm an expert in what my own body needs, there are thousands of ways to be disabled. I don't have the lived experience to navigate the finer points of what someone with low vision or limb difference or dwarfism needs, but behind the scenes, the staff at Nikki Ray are doing their utmost to skill up. They hire a disabled intern and we all participate in Integrated Described Video training, courtesy of AMI.

I share what I know with the team. I deem Stella Young's TED Talk on "Inspiration Porn" to be required viewing. I recommend Rebekah Taussig's memoir, *Sitting Pretty,* and Alice Wong's anthology, *Disability Visibility*. None of these are textbooks for how to make a film set inclusive and accommodating, but they do provide insights on how to not be weird, and not being weird to the show's disabled cast and makeover candidates is crucial to the success of the show.

Nailing the tone of the show is equally critical. There can be no sad soundtracks, no B-roll hospital footage. This is not a campaign that pimps out the sick to raise money or awareness for charity. *Fashion Dis* isn't here to fix anyone, because nobody is broken. Our goal is to create magazine-quality images of disabled fashionistas and to showcase adaptive fashion, beauty trends and technology that address the sartorial needs of people who don't want their prosthetic leg fucking up the drape of their pants. *Fashion Dis* exists so that people who have never seen the aspirational versions of themselves in media can find the style role models we all deserve.

Our makeover participants are welcome to share as much or as little of their medical histories as they want, but for the purpose of the show, we will be identifying each person by their name, not their disability. As Cara says, "If I have trouble finding clothes that fit because I've gained weight, you don't need to know why I gained weight. It's nobody's business." It's the same with disability. If using a wheelchair means I need pants with a higher rise in the back, I can explain why a higher rise is more comfortable without explaining why I need a wheelchair (though it should be obvious that I don't want to expose the crack of my ass).

As supportive as the producers are, I have to consciously, and repeatedly, decide not to receive accommodations for me or for any of the show's disabled participants as charity. Still, I try to be easy to work with. There are a lot of people trying to bust into the entertainment industry, and I let it slide when my quiet dressing room gets taken over by hair and makeup, or when the path to the couch becomes storage for half a dozen tripping hazards. Disabled or otherwise, we are all victims of the cult of productivity. These are honest oversights, and I don't want to pull any diva bullshit. Frankly, it's hard enough to ask for accommodations the first time. Ask again for the same thing and it can feel like you're asking for too much.

When I'm feeling a little too extra, I remind myself that without the disabled community, there is no show. That we are the assets, not the problem, and I try to adopt the Big Dick Energy of Zach Anner, one of my favourite disabled actor/writer/creators, who somehow manages to be incredibly humble and generous and joyful while leading with the knowledge that, no matter what the accommodations, he brings something to the table that benefits the rest of the people in the room, that the people who have facilitated his access are the lucky ones because he is there sharing his brilliance.

Ardra Day happens toward the end of a month of filming, and part of what makes saying "I'm Ardra Shephard" feel so damn good is how proud I am of the work I've done so far, and how grateful I am to my body for its relative compliance—for actually letting me pursue this incredibly rare and extraordinary opportunity to influence the culture. It's been a dream come true. In fact, the only really hard day was the first day.

In a past life, spending two hours trying on clothes would have been time well spent at the "good" mall with my BFF, Tracy. For various reasons, my wardrobe fitting got bumped, and then it got bumped again until it could get bumped no more, and we had to fit in the fitting the day before we started filming. This, incidentally, was three hours before my one and only on-set rehearsal. We had two hours to come up with seven looks despite the fact that it takes me four full minutes just to put on socks. I don't think I was taken seriously when I said, "However long you think it takes me to get dressed, triple it."

The fitting was at the cool but woefully un-air-conditioned studio of designer and *Fashion Dis* wardrobe expert Izzy Camilleri. It was a warmer-than-usual September day that did nothing but slow down my already sluggish nerve conduction, but seeing dozens of hangers full of colour and textured fabric on a rack of clothes with my name on it produced enough adrenalin to help me power through the heat.

My weak arms and lack of core strength meant I occasionally got trapped in a dress or a sweater. My legs live by the mantra "we do what we want" (which means they do nothing). Lifting each leg into its pant leg opening with my aforementioned weak arms is like dressing a mannequin with the arms of another mannequin, and both mannequins are twice my weight. When we inevitably ran out of time, I was too weak to try on anything else anyway. I consented to a skirt that looked like it would fit, and said yes to a jumpsuit despite the fact that jumpsuits are the Olympics of dressing and a race against time whenever I have to pee, which would be often, because I had a UTI. (Of course I did.)

I arrived on set for my rehearsal certain that I was about to blow it before we'd even started. I was *Weekend at Bernie's*–level tired, but no one seemed to notice that I was legally, if temporarily, dead. I didn't say anything, but it did not, at that moment, feel particularly good to be Ardra Shephard.

Cara told me we'd film some mock interviews—no notes, no cue cards, just wing it—then watch them back in Video Village (more lingo; it's a room with a lot of screens) so I could see what I needed to work on before we started filming for real *the next day*. Super chill, right?

I interviewed Sam, one of the producers. I asked about her earliest style memory, what she thought her style says about her, if she'd ever felt dissed by the fashion industry. Sam answered honestly. She even got emotional.

"You got this, babe. You're ready," Cara says, after the interview. "I don't even want to show you the footage, because I don't want you to get in your head. Just keep doing what you're doing. It's great. *You're* great." I'm glad she thinks so. I have such high hopes for this show.

That disabled bodies deserve to be seen and celebrated is not even close to a universally accepted truth. Disability is part of who we are and what we do with our circumstances. Disability impacts all of us. When it's not a given that all bodies have equal and inherent value, we need to say it again, louder, and with sequins—until it sinks in.

50 / Amazing Grace

IT'S BEEN A WHILE since I've seen Darcy IRL. She bailed on my last two parties, and I hate going to the burbs. Then COVID hit, and texts and phone calls have been all either one of us has been able to manage. No worries. We have the kind of relationship where we can go ages without connecting, then pick up right where we left off. Which is great because we have a lot to catch up on.

The hot goss is that after doing hard time kissing frogs all over Southern Ontario, Darcy finally found her Prince Charming: a grade-A guy named Bobby who worships the ground she rolls on.

In 2022, Darcy agrees to come on my new podcast to talk about the difficult work of finding The One. She's ready to spill the tea on what dating is like as a wheelchair user with progressive MS: the good, the bad, the ugly—she saves the horrifying for me. Darcy wants to share her love story so that people with progressive MS and other disabilities can see what's possible, and know that dating is a shit show for everyone—disability or not—but that ultimately it's worth it.

The day of the recording Darcy joins the video call from a sunlit room in the lakefront condo she shares with Bobby. She's bothered by tinnitus, and the weakness in her hands made it difficult for her to put on makeup. It's the kind of frustrating shit that railroads me when I'm trying to get out the door, but Darcy doesn't seem rattled. Darcy's a natural beauty. Her dirty-blonde bob and cat-eye glasses make this former teacher look like a sexy librarian.

I introduce her on the show as "a real-life rom-com." Universal should secure the rights and put her story on the big screen. On the other hand, with all the drama, the intrigue, the alcohol that happens behind the scenes when you're dating with this disease, I feel like *The Real Housewives of MS* could also make a compelling addition to the reality franchise. If Universal passes, I'd watch the shit out of *that* TV show. (Andy Cohen, call me.)

When people ask who my MS role models are, I always name Darcy. Her MS has been more aggressive than mine. It often feels like Darcy's experience is a harbinger of what's coming for me.

"Is it fair to say, it's nice to meet the canary in Ardra's coal mine?" my podcast co-host, Alex, asks Darcy at the top of the show.

Ew. When Alex says it out loud, I suddenly feel uncomfortable about the pressure I'm putting on my friend who is sicker than I am, following her into a haunted house only as long as she can confirm that, yeah, there's a family of rats and some huge hairy spiders living in there, but the bogeyman is drunk and taking a nap.

Back in the day, Darcy would describe herself as a glass-half-empty kind of girl, and this perspective added to the appeal of making her the personification of reassurance. As more of a find-the-gratitude type, I believed that if Negative Nelly could still find joy in an increasingly disabled body, I could too.

When I was still shoving mobility aids out of pictures, Darcy told me that eventually that bullshit goes away. She doesn't lose any sleep stressing over her wheelchair anymore. "I know how tired you must be," she'd said, "and how sad you are. If you end up in a chair, you will be okay. You will still be the beautiful, brilliant, funny and amazing woman you are."

Other people have probably said some version of this to me, but Darcy is the only one with enough authority to make it believable.

Meanwhile, Darcy still cops to feeling jealous of seeing me on TV, standing upright, even if I am attached to a cane or a rollator. It stokes her anger at the course her disease has taken, before her feelings quickly turn to pride. We're still comparing ourselves to each other, and not to healthy controls, but we've grown up; we've gained considerable perspective.

Maybe Darcy's glass was half-empty back in her twenties. Who wasn't angsty then? Over the years, her glass seems to have gotten fuller, even as the circumstances around her MS have gotten harder. She's recently given up drinking, and become a wellness coach (the natural evolution of a suburban MLM enthusiast), but Darcy's joy was always there. And I've never been tougher than her, not even close.

One of Darcy's key messages about dating that she shares on the pod is that not everyone can roll with MS, and that's okay. At her core she believes that some people can, and do, and will. You just have to find the right person. She tells the audience, "I don't need to convince anybody of my worth. The people that are so supportive in my life, they're the people to focus on."

Preach.

"You have to not be afraid. You have to know that you will find it. Have faith and put in the work. If you really, really want to find that person, you can't give up." It's like the words are coming right out of Julia Roberts' mouth.

When Darcy talks about the frog who freaked out after they'd been dating for four months and she fell in the bathroom of a restaurant, she is full of life and wisdom. She tells the story like it's on him for losing his shit, because falls happen. Duh. It's not about her. He couldn't handle a little spilled milk. Darcy's sense of self-worth is so contagious that I immediately renew a promise to myself not to apologize for the next MS-related calamity or inconvenience in my own life, because MS is not my fault. (Easier said than done.)

After the recording, we debrief. "Did I seem nervous?" Darcy asks.

"You killed it. You were fab."

"That was the coolest thing ever," Darcy beams. "If it helps just one person, it will have been worth it."

"Are you kidding? You should write a book."

"You should write it," Darcy says. Then her tone shifts to something more confidential. "Things are getting bad, Ard. Like, really bad."

The medication that keeps Darcy's spasticity under control is no longer effective. She's getting a device, a baclofen pump, surgically inserted into her abdomen so that the drug can be delivered directly to the space around her spinal cord. Meanwhile, the pump will have a neighbour, because Darcy's hand has become too weak to manage self-catheterization—never mind applying mascara—so she's getting an indwelling catheter too.

Just hearing about these interventions forces my face to contort into a frown of empathetic discomfort. These invasive procedures—portals directly in and out of her body—are evidence that Darcy's MS is indeed getting harder, but Darcy spins them as solutions that make life easier, the shit we do to survive. What other choice does she have?

I'm bummed to hear that Darcy's MS sucks more than ever, but it's not surprising. How many times have we borne the unbearable? Too many to count. MS gets harder. That's MS's MO. It's not easy to tell from the outside when things have gone from bad to worse to worst. Still high from our interview, I focus on the bright light she was on the show. I take Darcy's medical update in stride, like the way TB didn't look up from his laptop last week when, after asking where I would like to be set up with my coffee, I said, "Six feet underground." When something is always the matter, it's hard to sound an actual alarm.

LATE ONE NIGHT, while TB and I are streaming *The Righteous Gemstones*, my phone pings.

"Who's texting you at this hour?" TB asks with a raised eyebrow, like I might have a secret lover.

"It's Darcy," I say. The only "u up?" texts I ever get come at ten in the morning from my mother, wanting to know if I'm literally awake. "She says she needs to talk, and that she could use my thoughts."

Never one to leave an SOS on "read," I text right back to let her know I'm around for whatever she needs. I make a mental note to mention all the positive feedback I'm still getting about the podcast. She's definitely helped more than one person.

Darcy doesn't reply until the next day, when she tells me she can't talk, because there are contractors in the house. Instead, she texts me that her symptoms are getting pretty unbearable. She's exploring end of life.

The information stops me cold. End of life? I'm baffled. It's only been six months since she was on the podcast, when she seemed to have had plenty of reasons to live. I'm almost more confounded by the presence of the contractors. I don't know how serious Darcy is, thinking about the time she has left, but I don't think she should have to spend any of it in the presence of fucking contractors.

My heart is racing. It's absurd to receive this kind of intel in a text, but I'm grateful not to have to process Darcy's bombshell in real time. Whatever the expression on my face is, I'm glad Darcy doesn't have to see it.

I need time to process, but I don't leave her hanging. I text right back, saying, "Fuck this disease. When can I call? I love you, Darcy. Can I come see you this weekend?"

Her text back simply says: "Yes."

"Maybe she wants you to talk her out of it. Didn't she say she wanted to know your thoughts?" TB asks as we try to guess at what the fuck is going on.

"What if she wants me to talk her *into* it? I'm not usually the person you call when you wanna be talked out of stuff. I'm more of the let-me-help-you-rationalize-a-questionable-decision type of girl. I don't, however, look forward to examining the ways in which this decision makes sense.

As the weekend approaches, Darcy texts to say she's not up for visitors after all. When I finally get her on the phone, I realize this is all very real. Darcy doesn't want my counsel, she wants to say goodbye. In addition to the recent developments of the catheter and the pump, Darcy must suffer the indignity of having a nurse come to her home, slap on a glove and digitally dis-impact her bowels every couple of days. But the sudden return of trigeminal neuralgia, an incredibly painful symptom, is the last straw on a pile of straws. If straw was made of red-hot pokers.

Darcy's doctor is keeping her comfortable. Ish. With meds. She needs something stronger. I tell her that now would be a good time to experiment with propofol. That the propofol nap is the only reason I'd even consider another colonoscopy. (Which is not an endorsement of recreational propofol. This is the drug that killed Michael Jackson.) I'm just saying there's a time and a place. Darcy laughs because that's what we do. Then she asks me to spell *propofol* so she can ask her doctor about it tomorrow.

When Darcy tells me she's relieved that she won't have to turn fifty, I laugh again because I get it. We're both still a handful of years from the big five-oh, but I'm already freaked out about it. Darcy tells me that ending her life means she won't have to endure the discomfort of getting her baclofen pump changed and she sounds so truly relieved—almost joyful—and that's when I stop laughing. The pump is due to be replaced in June. It's March 19. I don't know what I thought, but this is happening too soon.

Except it's not too soon for Darcy. She's been thinking about MAID for years. Her family—Bobby, everyone—is supportive. "What about Grace?" I ask, thinking about her nineteen-year-old daughter.

"She's going to be mad, but she's going to be okay," Darcy says with a mother's knowing. Darcy is peaceful. Resolved. The only bitterness in her voice comes when she talks about Bobby.

"It feels cruel that I only just found him, and now I'm going to lose him," she laments. It is cruel. This disease is so fucking unfair. Still, I thank God for Bobby. If Darcy was alone, or lonely, I don't know if I could make peace with MAID being the right call on a decision I already suspect will haunt me.

"Besides narcotics, is anything bringing you comfort?"

"Bobby, the dog. We just finished watching *Your Honor*."

"What about food?" I ask.

"Every meal is dessert," she says. Darcy to the end.

We finish our call saying "I love you" instead of goodbye. I tell her to call any time at any hour, knowing she won't. It's easier to hang up pretending we'll connect again.

"I need you to go to Barber and buy out the entire shop," I tell TB. Barbershop Patisserie is my favourite bakery this side of France. Run by Jill Barber, a Paris-trained pastry wizard, she makes the best croissant in the city. You can get them only after 10 a.m., because the woman, God bless her, believes in sleep. She makes a lemon *bichon* that tastes like the sugar-torched top of crème brûlée, and a poached rhubarb on custard that is as pink and pretty as it is delicious. If I were dying, but still had a dessert tummy, I'd want a hundred dollars' worth of whatever Jill was baking that day.

Darcy isn't taking visitors, but I figure we could leave a package at the door. We drive to Burlington and drop off an enormous box of sugar and butter and love, and a card:

> *Brave, beautiful Darcy,*
> *Grateful isn't a big enough word for what your friendship, sense of humour, realness, wisdom and support have meant to me.*
> *I will never forget you.*

I stay in the car while TB takes the package to the concierge. It's too soon for me to know how I will possibly make sense of MS without Darcy. Or what Darcy meeting her threshold means for me meeting my own.

While I wait for TB to return, I notice a couple of guys in workwear having a cigarette next to their construction company van. They're wearing heavy boots and T-shirts, despite the fact that it's still jacket weather. Contractors. Are these the same guys who were working in Darcy's unit? Before my indignation at the decision to permit contractors anywhere near my friend can turn into full-blown rage, I consider that if there were indeed renovations happening in Darcy's apartment (as opposed to some kind of plumbing emergency, in which case I withdraw my objection), she probably made the arrangements herself. Darcy is practical. Darcy is a decision-maker. Darcy is in charge. Investing in renos and repairs, making a home more comfortable, more beautiful, more livable is ultimately an act of optimism. It's the kind of thing someone who, even at the end of her own life, does knowing that somehow, impossibly, life will go on without her.

RIP, Darcy Zelinksy
September 10, 1977–April 12, 2023

51 / Here We Are

"I'M FALLING IN LOVE WITH THE BANKER," Wendy says.

"It's like he walks around with a halo," Suranjita adds.

"Does he have a brother?" Shannan wants to know.

It's Wednesday night, which means I'm at my writers' group, Write Club (we're less violent than *Fight Club*, but just as exclusive). I've just read the latest chapter of my in-progress memoir (the one you're reading now), and these drooling vultures need to settle the fuck down. The Banker's not on the market. My toes may be blue and my baseline body temp sub-vitally cold, but I'm not dead yet.

I'm not even actively dying, though I am a little obsessed with my own mortality lately. It doesn't help that in addition to a recent diagnosis of something called geriatric rhinitis, I can now add osteoporosis to the list of conditions nudging me toward an early grave. My old-lady bones made themselves known after a fall from standing, wherein I fractured my delicate spine, presumably thanks to years of IV steroids. So this, too, is on MS.

I'm anxious to get on treatment to stop my cannibalizing body from sucking dry what's left of the calcium in my skeleton, but my doctor is reluctant to prescribe the monoclonal antibodies that help restore bone density, because there's a limit to how long you can take them.

"It's not like I'm going to live to be eighty," I'd said to my doctor, surprised by the foreboding words coming out of my mouth. I (more than) half expected her to refute my claim, to tell me I was being preposterous (like when you ask your bestie if your peplum top makes you look like a penguin in a tutu, and she says, "Of course not, you look fab," even though peplum looks good on nobody).

When my doctor didn't dispute my grim prediction and told me she would send me to a specialist instead, I interpreted her blow-off as medical confirmation that my shortened expected lifespan is not something I just made up—that I have, in fact, been put on the fast track to heaven.

I don't know how long I think I'm going to live, or exactly how many of those years will be "good" ones. I have a guess, but even I know better than to put it in writing. The point is, I don't need to protect Octogenarian Ardra, I need to protect forty-something Ardra. I need to look out for Ardra Now. When I think about how I'm willing to roll the dice on bone drugs, I start to wonder why I'm stressing about the long-term use of zopiclone when I could be getting consistently better sleep. Why am I worrying about anything? According to my last credit card statement, if I pay the minimum, it will take forty-eight years and four months to pay it off. That is a tempting offer, Visa. Thanks for doing the math.

I mention my prognosis to Tracy, the same bestie whose job it is to unquestionably support temporary insanities, like my brief exploration of peplum. When I quote the doctor, I use my "how dare she?" voice. But all Tracy hears is a call from The Future: *Ring, ring, some day your best friend is gonna die! Time to start thinking about that!*

I'm shocked when she starts to cry, before pulling herself together.

"I guess I'll have to look after TB," she says, in an attempt, I guess, to be helpful.

"Fuck that guy!" I say, trying to lighten the mood. "He'll be sad for a while. Devastated. But eventually, he'll be okay. All this hair, good job, no kids, grieving widower *with a car*? Your job will be to keep the vultures away."

Clearly I'm having a mid-life crisis. I don't need to buy a new car or have an affair. (Though I could use a mini disaster to rationalize the Ami Paris bag I've been eyeing.) I've already lived a good life, done some cool, and even meaningful, shit. I'm proud of the life I've lived and grateful for the experiences and opportunities I've had. Getting sick early in life means I've been adjusting my priorities for decades, so there's nothing major to reassess. I don't love what's going on with my sagging ass, but I realize that literally no one else cares. There are things I still want to do, of course, but if I never make it to Japan, whatever. Toronto has decent sushi, and if wasabi Kit Kat was any good, it would be available at Shoppers Drug Mart by now. I'm not a total mid-life cliché. It's just that, holy shit, we're all gonna die someday, a fact that's starting to feel more true than it used to.

Meanwhile, a significant chunk of my peer group is about to turn fifty. These are the people who should be having mid-life meltdowns, but everyone seems so chill about fifty, excited even. They're planning trips and parties, investing in "Fab at Fifty" regimens that include yoga, cardio and juicing. They are motivated to get in the stronger-than-ever, best shape of their lives, like fifty doesn't have a downside. Thanks to Gwyneth and Drew, even menopause seems to be having a sexy pop-culture moment. My friends are all so certain that the best is yet to come. I still have a few years before the big five-oh, so it's not up to me to tell them it gets worse—they'll figure that out on their own.

As it happens, TB is one of the first in our circle about to hit the half-century mark, though he hasn't hopped on the "Fab at Fifty" trend, thank God. He's not rubbing the joys of aging in my geriatric-rhinitis-riddled face. Oh sure, he walks to work and takes a probiotic, but his wellness plan is mostly limited to Dry February (it's the shortest month of the year) and being genetically thin. Turning fifty isn't going to stop his daily visits to the candy bar in the break room at the bank, or make him consider getting more than five and a half hours of sleep. He shrugs off fifty, claiming, "It's just a number," as if numbers are neutral (ask him how he feels about the number attached to the credit card I decided I no longer have to pay). Still, I know his birthday needs to be special, that it should stand out from the rest, and so we decide to spend it in New York City, where we can catch a couple of shows, see the Tiffany reno, visit our favourite paintings at the MoMA, spend some face time with Mike and his girls.

I book the nicest hotel we can afford, knowing I'll spend half our waking hours resting. A room with a view, a rooftop bar, a strategic location: we check into a hotel close to trendy East Village shops and restaurants, around the corner from the famous Strand Bookstore. My love for travel used to feel like part of my identity, but FOMO tends to fade in direct relation to how desperate I am to just lie down, and I dread the day when I start to feel like the inconvenience and discomfort of MS makes travel no longer worth it.

While I'm sacrificing a lot, I feel even more bummed about the things my MS makes TB miss out on when we're on vacation. TB doesn't exude long-suffering vibes. My guilt is self-manufactured. In general, TB insists he isn't missing anything, and that without me, he'd still be watching TV in his parents' basement, eating Subway on special occasions. He believes he never would have set eyes on the Louvre, watched *Aïda* under the stars in Verona, tasted pigeon in Scotland or paella in Spain without me to lead the way. But I think he chose me because, on some level, he was looking for these experiences. If I hadn't been the one to expand his horizons, he would have found someone with similar qualities.

Which isn't to say I think I'm replaceable. Not even close. The Banker is a devoted and sentimental dude. Our first dog together, our cherished doodle Rihga, lived a long doodle life. She's been gone for more than four years now, and every morning when he leaves for work, TB gently touches the photo of her that hangs by the front door.

I loved that bitch like I had personally birthed her, but it didn't take long for our replacement dog, Tilly, to fill the Rihga-sized hole in my heart. Meanwhile, TB remembers Rihga with rose-tinted glasses. He forgets the times she barfed in the car or chewed the leg of the couch. Of course TB loves Tilly, probably more than he realizes, but Tilly will never be Rihga, and I think he sometimes holds it against her.

I take some consolation in knowing that once I'm a dead ghost, all the annoying shit I do will be forgotten too. I've never barfed in the car, but I have wrecked some furniture. I've definitely broken some dishes. I can't imagine my ghost will need TB to touch my picture on his way out the door every day, when once a week seems reasonable. Like Saint Rihga before me, there will be no living up to Saint Dead Wife.

IT'S NEARING THE END of TB's birthday trip to New York and we've just come from a posthumous production of Sondheim's final work, *Here We Are*, a musical where the music drops dead two-thirds of the way into the show, possibly because Sondheim, who lived to be ninety-one, didn't live long enough to finish the score. It's a beautiful production of a purgatory that does nothing to lessen my running-out-of-time concerns, let alone the feeling that life's too short for all of us—that in the end (and even in the beginning, and the middle sometimes), we're all basically doomed.

Again, I am not actively dying, but The Banker's fiftieth birthday is jacking up my anxieties about not just his life, but about *ours*. We've known each other for twenty-six years now—more than half my life. It's one thing to pass through the middle point of "me," but thinking about the halfway mark of "us" makes it difficult to breathe. I am feeling extra emotional and dramatic, so let's see where that takes us.

"What if the time we've already had together is greater than the time we have left?" I'm dropping a bombshell, but just like my doctor, and Tracy, The Banker doesn't protest.

"We've done so much already," he says. "We saw two shows, hung out in Washington Square Park, had dinner under the Brooklyn Bridge. I talked to David Hyde Pierce today."

"That dinner was freezing." (We ate outside because I'm still not taking any chances with COVID.) "As for DHP, he said thanks after you threw five bucks in the Broadway Cares bucket."

"And I said, 'You're welcome'!"

"Anyway, I'm not talking about this trip," I say. "I feel like I'm running out of time. Time with you."

"Sheppy, we've already done more than I ever thought I would," he says, again, as if everything we've already had has been enough. I don't bother criticizing his lack of imagination.

"Are you saying we had a good run?"

"I'm saying everything else is gravy."

I steel myself, then say what's been on my mind a lot lately: "One day, when I'm gone, you're going to have this whole new chapter, this whole other life without me. You'll still have time to do the things we can't do together." I choke on the words, but I mean them generously, or at least without bitterness. My self-indulgent absolution relieves me of my guilt when I think about the limitations MS imposes on our life. That there is an "After Ardra" is the consolation prize that's meant to close the gap between the highs and lows, the sacrifices and the benefits of being with me. I know I'm worth it, but it's fucked up that my brain actively has to point it out, that I have to remind myself that I was the logical choice for The Banker's life when he has so obviously been the logical choice for mine.

Dying wishes are manipulative and unfair. We don't owe anything to the dead. Once again, I'm not technically dying, but if I *were* dying, my wish for TB—in the spirit of sometimes knowing what's good for him more than he knows himself—would be for him to always have a dog. I feel like he would figure the rest out himself, but I continue to pitch him the perks of the After Ardra anyway. "You could travel to places with extreme spiders, go camping, find a replacement wife who actually likes sports. Maybe she has kids. You'd be a great stepdad."

"I'll grow a beard for a year," he says, without even commenting on my endorsement of a replacement wife. Like he's also thought about the After Ardra, considered his grieving process, put a time limit on it and knows what costume he'll wear. This is the part in the script where he's supposed to say he could never go on without me, and that if I want to be buried in peplum, so be it. Forget about a grief beard; he'll spend a year wearing peplum himself.

"What happens after a year? You shave your beard and hop on Tinder?"

"My beard would be crazy after a year," he says reflectively, like a grief beard is some kind of hair shirt. Like this motherfucker doesn't hate shaving. Talk to me when you give up eating candy from the break room.

"What the hell? I want you to be okay *eventually*. You're not supposed to realize that life goes on without me until long-the-fuck-*after* I'm dead." Benevolent Ghost Wife has left the chat. I am no longer full of wisdom and grace. I've moved on from freaking out about running out of time to freaking out about why he's not freaking out too. Happy birthday!

"Why aren't you having a mid-life crisis?" *j'accuse.*

"Why are *you*?" he asks.

"Because fifty, and MS, and climate change, and the collapse of democracy, and the robot zombie apocalypse. Because everyone I know and love will someday die. Because Darcy. Because here we are and the sky isn't falling, but it's definitely starting to crumble." There's something tempting about touching a hot stove, about standing on a subway platform and thinking about what it would be like to get hit by a train before stepping back and retreating to acceptable human behaviour.

"Sheppy, you are not Darcy," TB says, finally turning serious, finally saying something I need to hear. I start crying in earnest. He hugs me, his body absorbing some of my meltdown, but even hugs have become a diluted version of what they once were. Something I can only partially participate in. Without strong legs or balance, I'm too weak for hugs to last as long as I need them. When moving my body even slightly takes so much effort, hugs are hard to initiate—hugs need to come to me.

"I don't need a mid-life crisis because I love our life. I'm not missing anything," TB says quietly into my ear.

"Don't you worry about when it ends? When it all goes away?"

"No. My life started with you. I don't think about a life without you. I can't. I won't."

Here we are indeed. Alive right now, together. Just trying to be here. And yet, here we go.

52 / Happy Endings

HOW MANY TIMES have I asked myself "how will I?" and answered "I just will"? Being diagnosed with MS is a big fucking deal, and from time to time I deserve to pay tribute to that. To say, *Holy eff, that happened to me.* Someone should buy me a present. I deserve so many presents, in fact, that I should get to register for big-ticket items at Holt Renfrew. Every day should feel like my birthday.

On the other hand, it's hard to congratulate myself for having gone through something when I haven't yet made it to the end. I'd love to Nora Ephron the rest of my story and insist on a happy ending, but the problem with happy endings is that we're rarely at the end. My life isn't over, I'm still in the middle, where things get worse, until they get better, until they get worse again, until they get better—repeat until the end of time.

MS gets harder, but it also gets easier. Figuring out how to live with this version of MS lets me believe that whatever this disease throws at me, I'll figure out how to live with that too.

Except for the inconvenience of brain damage, my life, so far, has turned out a lot like I dreamt it would. A loving partner, a condo in the sky, creative work, ride-or-die friends, a couple of dogs, trips to Paris, a killer wardrobe, great skin. I might not be a singer, but the details don't matter. I love and am loved. I have purpose.

What's best about my life is also what makes it the most painful, knowing I could lose anything at any time. When good things happen, asking myself "if this is possible, what else is possible?" can be a comforting contemplation. But when bad things happen, the same logic can suddenly feel like a threat. Peace means surrendering to living in the sublime, before one thing becomes something else. Life's only certainty is change. There is no new normal, only the next normal and the next normal after that.

It's just after 9 a.m. and I don't have to put on a bra or pants for my 10 a.m. Zoom. I don't even have to put on deodorant. No one can smell my hair through the internet, but I should brush my teeth, grab a clean shirt and take my meds, plus I definitely need coffee, so I reluctantly decide it's time to get out of my cozy bed.

I start to rouse, making very little noise, but even from two rooms away, our doodle Tilly, who is perpetually on high alert for signs of life, takes notice. Any indication that I am remotely conscious is interpreted as an invitation to party. Still on my back, I start to take off my night-time ankle orthotic when the sudden and furious sound of tap dancing on hardwood announces the dog's imminent arrival.

Before I can grab the second orthotic, Tilly crosses the threshold to the bedroom and does an Olympic-length long jump, her bum moving vigorously left to right like a propeller while her body flies through the air. She sticks the landing in the centre of the bed, then drapes her panting enthusiasm across my chest, TB trailing behind her.

"No!" I cry, as fifty-four pounds of muscle and fur overwhelm me. Tilly's long pink tongue tries to cover me in kisses. I bring my hands up to protect my face. "No kisses!" I plead through my fingers, but I can't stop laughing as she licks my hands, her tail thumping the bed beside me in an unbridled declaration of how fucking fantastic it is to be alive. I bury my face in the pillow but TB has decided to get involved, and lifts up my T-shirt, offering Tilly a patch of stomach to bless with her big, sloppy mouth instead. The Banker's involvement means it's time to move on from kisses. It's time to play and Tilly slaps her paws on my chest.

Tilly has no idea that MS is terrible, that life in general is fucking terrible. Despite all the pain and suffering that comes with being alive, surely it's some kind of miracle that we humans are also built for joy.

Tilly is anxious for me to get up so that we can start the day, because, without any evidence to back up her thesis, she is certain that it's going to be a great day, possibly the best day of our whole goddamn lives. And what do I know? Maybe she's right.

ACKNOWLEDGEMENTS

WHEN I TOLD MIKE I was writing a book, his eyes shot wide open and he asked if someone was helping me. "What, like my *mom*?" I scoffed. But actually, my mom did help. She helped me a lot. Thank you, Norma Shephard, for reading every word, for policing my grammar, for laughing at my jokes and for championing and cheerleading almost everything I do, whether in life or on the page.

Thank you to my creative mentors, John Fanning, Barbara Radecki and Andrew Morris. To the women of Write Club, thank you for your consistently on-point insights and enthusiastic support. Thank you, Marie Gaudreau, for your tireless work translating *Tripping on Air*, bringing my voice to a francophone audience.

Kari Babinetz, without you this book could have been a horror story instead of the love story it is. To everyone else I adore and wrote about—Jim Shephard, Corinne Kramer, James Shephard, Mike Beck, Tracy McKenzie, Laura Hillyer, Sherry Charlton, Sammy Davis, Val Spironello, Imre Olah, Kevin Mallon, Jenny Angus, Lisa Hegedus, Heidi Webber, Alex Hajjar and Leigh Pettipas—thank you in advance for your grace at being included in my version of events, and if I didn't get it right, I blame MS.

Grace Hewitt, your mother was so proud of you. If you ever happen to read this book, I hope it gives you the chance to hear her voice again.

To the medical professionals tasked with the impossible job of keeping me in good health, in particular: Dr. Raymond Lo, Dr. Sharon Grad, Dr. Jiwon Oh, Dr. Armistead Williams, Dr. Marc Fischer, and the BARLO MS Centre. Thank you for your humanity and for genuinely caring about me.

Thank you, Ariel Brewster, Anna Comfort O'Keeffe, Larissa Giroux, Kelly Jones, Emma Skagen, Naomi MacDougall, Emmy Nordstrom-Higdon and Jake Babad for making it possible for me to say, "Holy shit, you guys, I wrote and published a book."

Finally, thank you to my younger self for keeping the diaries that helped inform these pages, and most importantly, thank you, Trippers, for tripping through life with MS and with me.

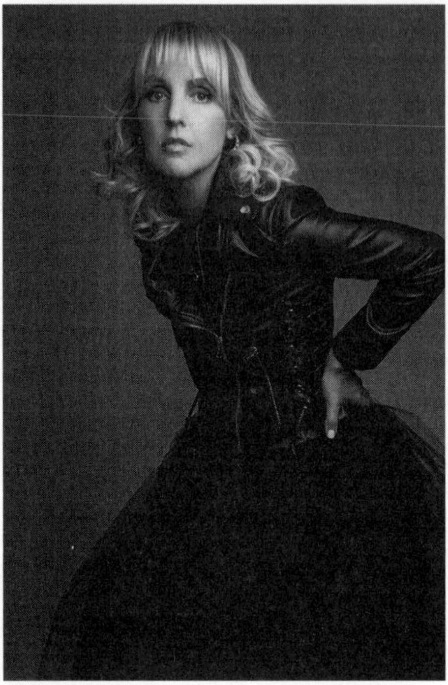

ALKAN EMIN

ABOUT THE AUTHOR

ARDRA SHEPHARD is a writer, consultant, podcaster and speaker whose award-winning blog, *Tripping on Air*, has an international reach and reputation. She is the creator and host of AMI-tv's lifestyle series *Fashion Dis.* Her personal essays and non-fiction work have appeared in *FASHION*, *InStyle*, *Best Health*, *BezzyMS* and other magazines and online publications. Ardra lives in Toronto, ON.